Health Essentials

Homeopathy

Peter Adams is a Registered Homeopath who has been practising for twelve years. He is joint owner of Stroud Natural Health Clinic in Gloucestershire, where twelve alternative/complementary medical systems are provided. His second book, *The Soul of Medicine* will be published by Penguin Books in 1997.

The Health Essentials Series

There is a growing number of people who find themselves attracted to holistic or alternative therapies and natural approaches to maintaining optimum health and vitality. The *Health Essentials* series is designed to help the newcomer by presenting high quality introductions to all the main complementary health subjects. Each book presents all the essential information on each therapy, explaining what it is, how it works and what it can do for the reader. Advice is also given, where possible, on how to begin using the therapy at home, together with comprehensive lists of courses and classes available worldwide.

The *Health Essentials* titles are all written by practising experts in their fields. Exceptionally clear and concise, each text is supported by attractive illustrations.

Series Medical Consultant
Dr John Cosh MD, FRCP

In the same series
Acupuncture by Peter Mole
Alexander Technique by Richard Brennan
Aromatherapy by Christine Wildwood
Ayurveda by Scott Gerson
Chi Kung by James MacRitchie
Chinese Medicine by Tom Williams
Colour Therapy by Pauline Wills
Flower Remedies by Christine Wildwood
Herbal Medicine by Vicki Pitman
Kinesiology by Ann Holdway
Massage by Stewart Mitchell
Reflexology by Inge Dougans with Suzanne Ellis
Self-Hypnosis by Elaine Sheehan
Shiatsu by Elaine Liechti
Natural Beauty by Sidra Shaukat
Spiritual Healing by Jack Angelo
Vitamin Guide by Hasnain Walji

Health Essentials

HOMEOPATHY

Natural Medicine
for the Whole Person

PETER ADAMS

ELEMENT
Shaftesbury, Dorset ● Rockport, Massachusetts
Brisbane, Queensland

First published in Great Britain in 1996 by
Element Books Limited
Shaftesbury, Dorset SP7 8BP

Published in the USA in 1996 by
Element Books, Inc.
PO Box 830, Rockport, MA 01966

Published in Australia in 1996 by
Element Books Limited
for Jacaranda Wiley Limited
33 Park Road, Milton, Brisbane 4064

Cover design by Max Fairbrother
Page design by Roger Lightfoot
Typeset by Footnote Graphics
Printed and bound in Great Britain by
Biddles Ltd, Guildford & King's Lynn

British Library Cataloguing in Publication
data available

Library of Congress Cataloging in Publication
data available

ISBN 1-85230-879-6

Note from the Publisher

Any information given in any book in the *Health Essentials* series is
not intended to be taken as a replacement for medical advice. Any
person with a condition requiring medical attention should consult a
qualified medical practitioner or suitable therapist.

Contents

Acknowledgements and Dedication

I would like to thank everyone who helped with this book. The many people I am grateful to include:

- patients who allowed use of their case-notes;
- the friends who commented on the manuscript, especially Hugh Barton, Paul Ingrams, Shauna Rammage and Michael Spalton;
- the homeopaths Julian Carlyon, Rissa Carlyon, Simon Eiles and Joy Adams and members of my family Eve, Fay and Grace who commented on the manuscript;
- Anja Liengaard who introduced me to homeopathy by treating Bessie the cow;
- Paul Jackson of Original Business Systems has given generously of his time and expertise;
- Sue Limb for the foreword and Julia McCutchen at Element Books for giving me the opportunity to write.

Finally I thank my family for giving me the time, and my parents for being my parents. This book is dedicated to them, Margaret and Ralph.

Foreword

DULCIE DOMUM TAKES HER DAUGHTER TO A HOMEOPATH.

'So: how are you Dulcie?'

'Oh, I'm fine, but Harriet's got a terrible cough. Sounds like a lorry load of coal being delivered. The doctor says linctus is useless and I'd just better reconcile myself to an awful winter.'

'Why don't you get real and go to a homeopath? Honestly!'

Alice hangs up – always a relief.

Ponder idea of homeopath. Have never liked the sound of it. Cross between homicide and psychopath. Still, nothing ventured, etc. Seize the free trade ads as recommended by numerous actors on TV 'Let your fingers do the walking.' – But what if your damned fingers can't walk either?

Arrive at natural health clinic. Heart sinks. Harriet writhes about jabbering. Heart sinks deeper. Homeopath however seems more interested in her behaviour than disapproving of it.

Harriet is questioned about her health, her history, the sort of weather she likes, the sort of food she likes ('Chips with vinegar') and what she wants to be when she grows up ('A Princess!'). He makes notes. Suspect his diagnosis is 'Mrs Domum cannot control her child who is a spoilt brat.' Discover later he is arriving at the conclusion that Harriet is a phosphorus type. This would explain why she fizzes about flashing and making a stink.

Once we have exhausted Harriet's history, though not her

hysteria, homeopath places a small pill on her tongue. Is that all? Unnerved by lack of linctus, bottles of pills, injections, elastic bandages, courses of physiotherapy, etc. Attempt to make further appointment. Homeopath assures me it's unlikely to be necessary.

Suspect he cannot face another exposure to my child, but two days later Harriet's cough, which had hitherto persisted three months, is completely gone.

The worst thing about going to the homeopath was Alice's triumph afterwards.

Sue Limb author of 'Dulcie Domum's
Bad Housekeeping' in *The Guardian*

Introduction

WITH THE HELP OF increased media coverage and public interest, homeopathy is taking a higher profile in our lives. A steady stream of TV and radio programmes and regular newspaper and magazine articles is appearing in response to increased interest in this system of complementary medicine. Sales of homeopathic medicines are increasing every year, and doubled in Britain between 1989 and 1994. A leading national pharmacy chain is now marketing its own brand in Britain. Homeopathy is definitely a growth area. In Europe during the 1980s its rate of growth was second only to the computer industry. The remedies are easy to use, which makes them popular in the home for first aid and for common illnesses. Private health insurance schemes are including homeopathy in response to increased public demand for professional homeopathic treatment for more serious problems.

Scientific and orthodox medical interest is growing, too. Articles on homeopathy appear more frequently these days in scientific and medical journals. More trials are being conducted demonstrating the effectiveness of homeopathic remedies for more and more diseases. A survey of trials of homeopathy published in the *British Medical Journal* in February 1991 concluded:

> The amount of positive evidence . . . came as a surprise to us. Based on this evidence we would be ready to accept that homeopathy can be efficacious, if only the mechanism of action were more plausible.[1]

There are many instances of sceptical doctors or medical researchers doing trials to demonstrate that homeopathy does not work, but getting unexpected results. They tend to conclude their research papers by saying that more research is needed and that an explanation must be found before homeopathy can play a larger role in our health care.

I understand this point of view very well because I subscribed to it myself until twenty years ago. I had a thorough academic education from Oxford University; Oxford was a stronghold of 'scepticism', a philosophical belief which says 'If something cannot be proved we cannot believe in it'. So when I went to a lecture on homeopathy in the early 1970s I rather ostentatiously walked out and thus made a statement about my sceptical attitude. 'It cannot possibly work! It is based on principles that are nothing more than nonsense.' However I was forced by the facts to change my mind.

A few years later I lived on a smallholding and had a sick cow. The veterinary surgeon could do nothing and there was a possibility that the animal would require an operation. A friend to whom I will always be grateful heard of our plight. She appeared with a little brown envelope containing some small round pills which she gave me with instructions on how to administer them to the cow. Those pills and those strange instructions will be familiar to many of you, but to me at that time they were an amusing eccentricity. I decided to go along with it, followed the instructions, and went to bed that night without thinking any more of it. The next morning I would have to make a decision. The digestive system of cows soon goes horribly wrong if they lie still for too long and my cow had been unable to stay on her feet for several days now.

The following day I went to the cow's open shed but she wasn't there. I looked out and saw her ambling slowly and peacefully across the field, grazing with that timeless pace cows have and giving the impression that there was nothing at all surprising about this. She needed a repeat dose of the remedy a few days later and another one after the next calving, but apart from that the problem, which was dislocation of the knee cap, never returned. (The remedy, by the way, was *rhus tox*.)

I could tell many more tales such as this. Although still unconvinced by homeopathic theory I was now intrigued. This seemed like magic. How did these little pills with hardly anything in them cure my cow, a beast totally immune to the placebo effect? I experimented with homeopathic remedies for the illnesses of my two small children. The success rate was high. Instead of wondering how it worked, I devoted myself to making it work even more successfully. When the treatments failed I went more deeply into the method of finding, for each case, the remedy that corresponded exactly to the illness. I became fascinated by the magic of homeopathy and went on to take professional training and set up my own practice.

When the extreme pain of a physical injury fades from your body after taking the remedy *arnica*, when you see your child's high temperature fall after taking *belladonna* (assuming it is the right remedy) you start to make your beliefs fit this new reality. People are rarely converted to homeopathy by an encounter with the theory. I certainly wasn't. But when it provides the solution in a time of dire need, or when it repeatedly does what it is not supposed to be able to do, then converts are made.

In their book on homeopathy, Dr Aubin and Dr Picard describe how they began their medical careers as orthodox general practitioners in rural France in the 1950s. One winter, one of their patients who had chronic bronchitis stopped needing antibiotics. They discovered that the patient was receiving homeopathic treatment and went to see the homeopathic doctor. They were impressed to learn that the method has a systematic clinical approach and is supported by a rigorous method of choosing the appropriate medicine; there are also many highly detailed reference books. They became homeopaths as a result of this experience.

Even though science has not yet found an explanation for it, homeopathy still succeeds in treating all kinds of medical problems. But how does it work? Scientists may be near to finding the answer.

The history of science is a history of expanding horizons; a continuous evolution of human understanding. At any point in time, it represents the limits of our vision rather than all there is to see.

> We continue to base our notions of health and illness, birth and death on visions of the world that have been transcended in our own time. . . . the very physics that we look to has been modified in this century in all its major facets. Thus we find ourselves with models in medicine that are characterized not by accuracy, as we wished, but by obsolescence.[2]

The science we are used to, the science that cannot explain homeopathy, is no longer the whole story. In the light of new discoveries the very dilute highly energized doses used in home-opathy are starting to make sense. In chaos and complexity theory very small changes in one part of a system can result in enormous changes elsewhere. This is what happens when a homeopathic remedy is taken. Our scientific understanding of the world is changing and the new theories are compatible with homeopathy.

These scientific revolutions are turning our understanding of the universe upside down. At the edges of our perceivable real-ity, that is, at sub-microscopic levels and at astronomical levels, reality becomes unreliable and the rules start to change. It is because homeopathic medicines are taken to one of these edges, the subatomic level, and brought back again, that they are so revolutionary.

If a system of medicine were to be created in accordance with the principles of new physics the result would be the reinvention of homeopathy. Chapter 3 will go a little further into the extraordinary support that is emerging for homeopathy from this physics. That 'plausible mode of action' may not be far away.

Proof of the effectiveness of homeopathy comes from many sources. In the appendix there are references to laboratory and clinical trials demonstrating that homeopathy really works, most of them published in medical journals. There are now millions of case records from all over the world confirming successful homeopathic treatments of all kinds of disease.

Part I

Understanding
Homeopathy

1
Understanding the Basics

WHAT IS HOMEOPATHY?

HOMEOPATHY IS A natural system of treating all kinds of illness. It is a subtle yet powerful system which works with the energies of life and produces genuine long-term cures in all kinds of illness. It has its own unique medicines, which are usually in the form of small, white, almost tasteless tablets. Like acupuncture and other similar methods of treatment, it is based on holistic principles. This means that the medicine treats the whole human being, not just one part or one disease. This is based on the belief that if one part is sick then this is the result of sickness of the whole person. As a result of putting the whole system back into balance, any disorder of an individual part of the body is put right from within.

Case Study
A teenager came to see me about his verrucas. After talking to him for an hour it was clear that he was, in homeopathic terms, a *natrum muriaticum* type. He hides his feelings, rejects sympathy if he is upset and has other characteristics of that constitutional type. During the first ten days of treatment with that medicine the verrucas fell out of his feet. Verrucas can only grow if the body allows them to. The homeopathic remedy puts the body back into balance, so that it eliminates the illness.

THE FOUR BASIC PRINCIPLES

There are four principles on which homeopathy is based. The first two are shared with other holistic health treatments:

1 The treatment stimulates the body's **natural healing power**. (In homeopathy this is called the *vital energy*.)
2 The treatment is **individually chosen** for each person.

The other two principles are unique to homeopathy:

3 The medicine is **similar** to the disease.
4 The doses used are minute and **potentized**.

We will now look at these principles more closely.

THE LAW OF SIMILARITY

The most important principle of homeopathy is the *law of similarity*. The word 'homeopathy' comes from two Greek words meaning 'similar suffering'. The law of similarity states:

> Whatever a medicine can cause in large doses in a healthy person, it can also cure in small doses in a sick person.

Put very simply, *like cures like*. The symptoms which a substance can cause can also be cured by it when it is given in the right way.

For example, arsenic causes diarrhoea and great weakness, accompanied by restlessness and anxiety. Yet homeopathic doses of arsenic have cured many people of this same condition, whether due to food poisoning, colitis or cholera.

So the first step in developing a homeopathic remedy is to find out what it can cause. A homeopathic medicine is taken by healthy human volunteers in repeated very small doses to discover the set of symptoms it creates. (The medicines are never tested on animals.) These tests are called *provings*. They are double blind, which means that neither the supervisor nor the volunteers know what the substance is, nor which volunteers are getting placebos. As soon as changes in the *provers'* state of health begin, they stop taking the medicine before any permanent changes are produced, such as the verrucas mentioned above. This ensures that the tests are safe. Each person's results

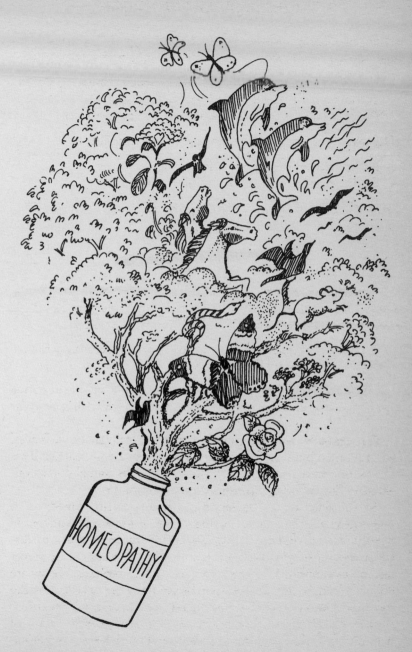

Figure 1   The homeopathic pharmacopea: all forms of creation can be made into medicines.

are recorded and these records are then used to make up the *materia medica*, a description of what that medicine can cause. This is also called the *remedy picture* of that medicine.

This information is then used when treating the sick, in the following way. All the symptoms experienced by the sick person are recorded and compared with the remedy pictures until a similar one is found. When this remedy is taken in a potentized dose it stimulates the body to heal itself.

These are some extracts from the proving of *arnica*, a plant which grows at high altitudes and is known as the 'fall herb':

> Internal pain as from a blow or a bruise. The nose pains from above downwards, as if he had had a severe fall upon it. In the cardiac region pain as if it was compressed, or as if it got a severe blow. Pain as from a sudden bruise. The arms are tired as if beaten.

The provers of *arnica* were getting symptoms normally associated with blows, falls and physical injuries generally. This guides us to its use: *arnica* is the main homeopathic remedy for all kinds of physical trauma.

EXAMPLES OF 'LIKE CURES LIKE'

When you peel an onion your eyes and nose run. Each time this happens it is a rudimentary proving of onion, *Allium cepa*. (Latin names are used for homeopathic remedies.) This means that *allium cepa* is one of the remedies used for colds and for hay fever where the eyes and nose run.

Case Study

A patient came to see me for homeopathic treatment because of panic attacks in the night which prevent him sleeping. He wakes suddenly at 1am, and is so restless he cannot stay in bed. He paces frantically around the house, and has such violent palpitations he thinks he is about to die. He is anxious, restless, cold and trembling until 3 or 4am. Sometimes he can get to sleep better if he goes to a different bed. This has all been worse since the threat of redundancy, which has led to great anxiety about his financial affairs.

Here are some extracts from the proving of arsenic, *Arsenicum album*, recorded by Dr Samuel Hahnemann, the founder of homeopathy, in his book *Materia Medica Pura*, published in 1830.

> About 1am excessive anxiety. He can find rest in no place, continually changes his position in bed, will get out of one bed and into another, and lie now here, now there. He is cold, shivers and weeps, and thinks in his despair that nothing can help him, and he must die. Violent palpitation in the night. Rambling at night.

The remarkable similarity between the panic attacks of the patient and the experiences of the provers of *arsenicum album* mean that *arsenicum* is the remedy for this man. Given in potentized form it prevented any more attacks for nearly two years.

THE BODY'S NATURAL HEALING POWER

The homeopathic medicine does not treat the illness directly, but enables the human body to do the necessary healing for itself. The focus is on the patient rather than the disease. Because the remedy is similar to the disorder it can stimulate the body to respond to the disease and cure it. Understanding this is crucial to the understanding of homeopathy as a whole.

If you get a throat infection, your body has allowed the bacteria to multiply in your throat. The homeopathic remedy will quickly stimulate your immune system to prevent this, and so deal with the infection.

In health, every moment of our lives, our bodies are keeping us free of disease by constantly adjusting and balancing all the activities of the body. We adapt successfully to environmental changes and psychological stresses and defend ourselves against bacteria and viruses. Living organisms have the natural power to maintain health built into them. We become ill only if our health maintenance system breaks down. Then we become *susceptible* to disease, and in order to be healthy again our defences need to be strengthened.

INDIVIDUAL TREATMENT

By treating the whole body, and its defences, homeopathy cures the illness. The medicine assists the forces fighting the illness so it has to be compatible with those forces. Each person's struggle against illness must receive exactly the kind of assistance it needs. The choice of medicine depends on the nature of the body's defences rather than the disease that is attacking it.

Case Study

A lady aged 35 needs treatment for ulcerative colitis which she has had since childhood. It was worse during pregnancy and since the birth of her twins eight weeks ago. She has been treated with intravenous steroids and other orthodox medicines. The diarrhoea contains a lot of blood and leaves her very exhausted, even to the extent that her speech becomes slurred and she becomes uncoordinated. Other problems have included acne, severe period problems and infertility. She also says she is a worrier.

The way her body is affected by the colitis, together with aspects of her personality, indicate that she is a *mercurius* type. This remedy had a wonderful effect on her, by stimulating her own defence mechanism. One month later the colitis was gone, she had reduced the steroids and expected to be off them the following week. She was much calmer, with a lot more energy and enthusiasm for life. Homeopathic treatment cures disease by strengthening the patient.

The way the body's defences are working is shown in the symptoms it produces in response to the disease. Two people with the same disease may not fight it in the same way and may therefore need different homeopathic treatment. For example, two people with hay fever may need different medicines. *Allium cepa*, the remedy mentioned above, is one of several possibilities.

How does the homeopath tell which medicine each person's *vital energy* needs? By studying that person and their individual symptoms in detail.

This is another central feature of homeopathy: *the medicine is individually chosen for each patient*. The homeopath carefully finds out about the whole person. The choice of remedy will depend not only on the physical symptoms the person has, but also on his or her state of mind.

Case Studies

Two children were brought to see me because of ear infections.

In the first case the pain had begun at 3pm the previous day, the right ear was hot and red, and the child had a high fever.

In the second patient the ear had a discharge with an unpleasant odour, and the child could not stand any coldness or the slightest touch in the region of her ear. The child was hypersensitive and irritable.

These two children had the same medical condition, but they were reacting to it in different ways. The remedy indicated by the first set of symptoms was *belladonna,* and by the second, *hepar sulph.*

POTENTIZATION

Nearly all homeopathic medicines are made from naturally occurring substances, mainly herbs and minerals. *Lycopodium* is made from the very fine spores of *clubmoss* which grows on remote heathland. *Drosera* is the insect-eating sundew plant. These are both herbs but homeopathy is distinct from herbalism because the medicines are diluted in a special way. They are diluted stage by stage until they contain extremely small quantities of the original ingredient. At the same time they are shaken, or *successed,* in a strictly controlled sequence. This process is called *potentization.*

Paradoxically, the most dilute medicines have the most powerful healing effect. Traditional science is unable to explain how such dilute doses can be effective, but several discoveries in new physics are starting to provide an explanation.

AN OVERVIEW OF THE HISTORY OF HOMEOPATHY

Although there are traces of homeopathic ideas right through medical history, homeopathy was only established as a medical system about 200 years ago, in Germany, by a successful doctor called Samuel Hahnemann. He had become thoroughly disenchanted with the primitive treatments then available and began doing his own research. His first momentous discovery was that when he took an overdose of a certain drug used as a malaria treatment, he got malaria symptoms. This was the first formal demonstration of the law of similarity.

After that discovery Hahnemann spent many years experimenting on himself and his students. They took repeated doses of many of the medicines of their day and recorded the effects very accurately. They ended the experiments before doing themselves any permanent harm. This was the first systematic programme of testing of medicines of any kind ever recorded. They continued this proving of remedies over many years and built up a record of the symptoms produced by these medicines which, because of the law of similarity, they could also cure. These remedies were then used to treat the sick. Sometimes treatments made patients worse, so smaller and smaller doses were tried. However, the small doses were less effective. In fact Hahnemann made little progress because the doses small enough to be safe were too small to be useful. It seemed impossible to make much practical use of the law of similarity.

Whether by accident or inspiration, Hahnemann then made his second great discovery – potentization. This special way of diluting medicines enabled him to make progress once more. He now had a method of making a medicine dilute enough to be safe, yet at the same time powerful enough to be effective.

By the early years of the 19th century the homeopathic method was established. The situation in medical circles was different in those days, and homeopathy was not seen at first as an alternative medicine. Many of the treatments used at that time were rather barbaric and people welcomed the gentle way of homeopathy. It spread rapidly across Europe and to the United States. Treatments were extremely successful, and the system was adopted by Queen Victoria. Ever since then the British Royal Family has used and supported homeopathy.

The most publicized success of the 19th century was in the cholera epidemics of the 1850s. When the death rates at the cholera hospitals were announced in Parliament in London the rates of the homeopathic hospitals were not included. But one MP insisted that the records be presented. They showed the extraordinary benefits of homeopathic treatment. In the homeopathic hospital in London 16.4 per cent of cholera patients died; elsewhere it was 51.8 per cent.

But the rise of homeopathy did not continue. As our present medical system grew stronger at the turn of the century, homeopathy went into a decline in the Western world which lasted until recently. Now homeopathy's fortunes are rising again as the limitations of conventional medicine become apparent. The demand for homeopathy is increasing dramatically and European manufacturers of homeopathic medicines regard Britain as a potential new market. Homeopathy is much more widely used in Europe. In France it is practised by 11,000 doctors and used by one third of the population.

WHAT IT IS LIKE TO HAVE HOMEOPATHIC TREATMENT

When you visit a homeopath, the first part of the consultation will be like a visit to your doctor. You tell the homeopath what is troubling you. But before long the direction of the interview will start to change. The homeopath will ask for apparently minor details of each symptom – such as the time of day when it is at its worst. Later there will be questions about you rather than your illness. For example, 'What are your favourite foods?' and 'Do you have any phobias?' The homeopath is building up a complete picture of you as well as your illness and of the less serious as well as the more serious problems. Equipped with knowledge of the homeopathic remedies, the homeopath will analyze these notes which may run to several pages. Then the homeopath can categorize you as a certain homeopathic type: perhaps a *nux vomica* or a *pulsatilla*. (These are the Latin names of two of the hundreds of different medicines used in homeopathy. Each one has been tested in a proving, as described in the last section.)

You will be given one medicine which will work on the whole of you: one medicine to stimulate healing even if you have several different complaints.

The medicine is usually given in the form of small, white, almost tasteless tablets. You will also be given instructions to avoid anything that antidotes homeopathy (see chapter 5).

You should then start to get better, possibly after getting

slightly worse. (In emergencies the homeopathic remedy will work very quickly and without an 'aggravation'.) The remedy initiates a natural healing process so, in long-term complaints, the improvement is often gradual. On the other hand it is not confined only to the main illness. You should feel better in yourself, be able to cope with stress better, and your health generally should benefit.

Initial consultations usually last from one to two hours and cost from 20 to 50 pounds in Britain. Further consultations cost less and are shorter and are rarely more frequent than once a month.

SOME COMMON MISCONCEPTIONS

'Homeopathy relies on the placebo effect'

It is sometimes suggested that homeopathic doses are so small that they cannot possibly work and that any benefits must be due to the placebo effect, or the healing effect of the long consultations. Homeopaths acknowledge that this may be true in any system of healing. However, the effects of homeopathy cannot be explained away so easily; they have nothing to do with suggestion or faith. The remedies work on animals, babies and patients who are unconscious. In these latter cases the patient is not even aware of receiving any medicine so the placebo effect can be discounted. Also, there may well be no consultation at all, so that explanation collapses as well. Here is a case where the patient was not aware of having homeopathic treatment.

Case Study
A distraught mother phoned me about her child, nine months old, who was teething. He was screaming inconsolably, and had to be carried around the whole time. After asking a few questions I told the mother to give the child *chamomilla granules*. The mother dropped a few into the baby's mouth. The baby hardly noticed, but a few minutes later stopped crying and fell into a peaceful sleep.

'Homeopathy is a form of vaccination'

The similarity between homeopathy and immunization is super-
ficial. They both administer a substance similar to the disease
and their effectiveness is based on their arousing a reaction to
that substance. Beyond that they are completely different.

Immunizations mobilize the healing forces of the body only
against one specific disease. Treatment with a homeopathic remedy raises the level of resistance to disease generally. The same
immunization is given to everyone. In homeopathy the treatment is individually chosen for each person.

Case Study

A man of 69 years visited my clinic just over a year ago.
Amongst other problems he was getting recurring colds, coughs
and flu. One winter he was laid low for months. For one year
after the treatment with his constitutional remedy, his immune
system was strengthened so that he was protected from all
previous illnesses.

'Homeopathy is unscientific'

To explain how homeopathy is scientific, it is helpful to distin-
guish between a scientific method and a scientific explanation.

Homeopathy is scientific in its method. The way of working
out which remedy to give is systematic and consistent. The
principles are clearly stated. The results can be assessed as in any
scientific investigation.

To be scientific, the question of an explanation for these
experimental results must be kept separate. Unbiased observation comes first. Only when we have the facts are we in a
position to start explaining them properly. More experiments
may then be needed. The controversial thing about homeopathy
is that the scientific explanation is incomplete. But the experimental results are still valid and await a full explanation. The
mechanics of the bumble bee's flight also await an explanation,
but its journeys from flower to flower continue. While the argu-
ment goes on, homeopaths continue applying their medical
methods scientifically to each case they meet.

Case Study

This is an example of a condition with no known cause or diagnosis, which responded to standard homeopathic treatment with the patient's constitutional remedy.

An elderly man wanted treatment for a pain in his right heel. Extensive investigations by several specialists and numerous tests over a period of two years could detect no abnormality. Several different medicines had been tried with no lasting effects. The pain was getting gradually worse so that he could now only walk for short distances. During the consultation it soon became clear that this man was a *lycopodium* type. For example he had abdominal distension and wind, usually worse between 4 and 8pm, and was allergic to onions. Psychologically, he was anxious when faced with anything new. All his life his greatest fear had been of public speaking.

Lycopodium cleared everything up, including his heel. A year or two later he came back for more *lycopodium* when the problems were starting to return.

PROFESSIONAL HOMEOPATHS AND HOMEOPATHIC DOCTORS

Once you have made the decision to have homeopathic treatment the next step is to find a properly trained homeopath. Although regulations in the British National Health Service have changed, most homeopathic treatment is still self-financed.

In Britain homeopathy is practised by some conventional medical doctors and by professional homeopaths. Professional homeopaths are regulated by the Society of Homeopaths. They usually work in natural health clinics or their own consulting rooms, and sometimes in GP's surgeries.

The Society of Homeopaths publishes the Register of Homeopaths which lists registered homeopaths in Britain. It also provides leaflets on homeopathy and other information. The Society is active in Britain and Europe in negotiating the future of professional homeopathy.

Generally speaking, professional homeopaths have more training in homeopathy and doctors have more training in medical science. Professional homeopaths tend to have longer consultations, although there are exceptions to this rule.

Doctors practising homeopathy are members of the Faculty of Homeopathy. The British Homeopathic Association provides information on homeopathy and lists of members of the Faculty.

TWO CASES WHICH SHOW THE WAY HOMEOPATHY WORKS

Case Study (Acute Treatment)

A female patient aged 32 phoned me on Christmas Day. She was seven months pregnant, and getting painful contractions, her abdomen is hard. The contractions are coming in quick succession, and are worse when she moves.

She was sixty miles away, visiting a friend for Christmas, but she managed to get the homeopathic remedy I suggested. It was also essential that she be admitted to hospital, where a fibroid tumour, grapefruit-sized, was discovered and thought to be the cause of the contractions. She left the hospital without any treatment the next day. She was a little better. Since the hospital could do nothing more we decided she should have another homeopathic remedy. I took down further details of her condition.

The pains are making her body tense up, and she is shaking and sighing and groaning involuntarily. The pains are of a tearing type and are made worse from any movement, even of the bed clothes.

There are two very meaningful homeopathic symptoms here: *the pains cause the patient to sigh, and uterine pains are made worse by movement.* These tell us about the state of the patient rather than the disease. They tell us what kind of healing measures the body is attempting and what kind of assistance the body needs in order to succeed in these attempts. Homeopathy enhances these attempts. The remedy for this case was *cimicifuga* and it worked very well. The contractions stopped over the next few hours and the patient soon felt well. After twelve days the fibroid could not be detected. A baby boy was born normally two months later.

This is an example of emergency treatment. The homeopath does not need to know about the constitution of the person. In treatment of acute conditions the 'here and now' symptoms are the important ones.

Case Study (Constitutional Treatment)

This is an example of a case where the curative remedy is selected mainly according to the personality type of the patient. All the other information is of less significance in the choice of the remedy.

A retired man, age 61, an ex-army officer was recommended to see me by his GP. He has had rheumatoid arthritis for ten years, especially in his hands. Penicillamine and injections of a gold compound helped a lot but he stopped them because of the side-effects. He now takes mainly anti-inflammatory drugs. He is always tired with aching pain in most joints, and a lot of stiffness. He cannot wear ordinary shoes. He gets flare-ups of the pain with fever.

So far the consultation has revealed an account of the disease diagnosis and allopathic treatment to date. With questioning from me, we now start to go deeper and record the information required for homeopathic purposes.

When the flare-ups happen the fever is accompanied by extreme chilliness; he shivers and sits in the corner next to the radiator wearing overcoats. The attacks start and end very suddenly.

He also has other problems; he takes Ventolin and Becotide for asthma which he has had since the age of three. The asthma and stiffness of the joints waken him at around midnight when he moves around for relief. All his life he has had a 'midnight feast' because he gets hungry at that time.

The asthma is made worse by sulphurous smoke, the smell of boiling fish and cigarette smoke. He never eats any fish because he gets swellings from contact. This first happened at the age of three when he nearly died.

We then went on to background personal information. He used to be badly affected by heat, for instance hot sunshine, but recently can stand sun better and has felt the cold more. He is an outdoor person and likes wild weather, but his hands get cold and his chest, strangely enough, gets hot. He has always been a sleepy person – embarrassingly, at any time. He is deeply refreshed by a short sleep of about twenty minutes. The foods he enjoys most are meat and vegetables.

He is afraid of the possible progression of the arthritis because he loves using his hands. He has virtually rebuilt the house and loves repairing things. Apart from this he confesses to being a bit idle, and his wife says he is very untidy.

Sulphur is a constitutional type well known in homeopathy as the 'ragged philosopher' or the 'absent-minded professor' or the 'eccentric inventor'. These people tend to be lazy about mundane things and untidy. They can easily take naps in the daytime and are very much refreshed by them. They get hungry during the night and can experience a sensation of heat of the chest. Clearly this describes the patient well, so I gave him homeopathic *sulphur* as his treatment.

At the follow-up appointment five weeks later he said he had been much improved for three weeks. Then he did some house improvements because he was so much better, and relapsed. But after a few days' rest he recovered again. He has put on weight. He had a cold that soon got better, which was a miracle because they usually sit on his chest for ages. He feels more alive and less tired by 30 per cent or more. The arthritis is 20 per cent better. In the past he has had bursae (fibrous lumps); one reappeared on his elbow and has disappeared again. His wife is convinced the homeopathic treatment has done him good.

He continued to make further improvements until he was almost entirely free of arthritic or other symptoms. From time to time he has needed repeat prescriptions of *sulphur*. Later, he incidentally revealed a little more of the characteristic *sulphur* inventiveness.

He is now able to wear normal shoes. Previous to the treatment he had only been able to wear trainers because of deformities of the feet due to the rheumatoid arthritis. He had invented his own shoe stretchers. He also adapted cutlery and hand tools.

This case contrasts sharply with the preceding one. The disease is long term (ie chronic). The homeopath focuses on the long-term symptoms and on the personality in order to decide on the remedy required.

WHAT TO EXPECT FROM HOMEOPATHY

The case above illustrates several important characteristics of homeopathic treatment for long-term illness:

1 In order to cure the disease it is necessary to treat the person. The remedy is chosen according to the personality of the patient and symptoms of the disease which are unique to that person; in the choice of remedy the disease diagnosis is of secondary importance.
2 When homeopathic treatment is working, past problems can temporarily reappear (in this case the bursae).
3 There is an improvement in the patient's well-being and energy as well as in the illness and this improvement often comes first.
4 Any other conditions that the patient possesses often benefit from the treatment (in this case the asthma, colds and loss of weight).
5 The patient continued to use the anti-inflammatory medicines until he no longer needed them. This is the general rule because most conventional medicines do not interfere with homeopathic remedies, and vice versa.

A person may go to a homeopath seeking help for arthritis. After asking about the problem and how it began, the homeopath will enquire about the person's state of mind, whether there is a problem with sleeping and much more. The treatment will be given for all these problems and at the follow-up appointment the homeopath will check on them again. Quite often the patient then realizes how many of the problems have improved under homeopathic treatment, even ones that were not mentioned initially.

Homeopathy has high expectations. In all but the most serious cases we aim to actually transform the whole organism so that it functions well in every way. At the end of the treatment you should be in good health and should stay that way without taking any medicine of any kind for long periods of time. You should feel balanced and positive. Diseased patterns are replaced by healthy ones. Homeopathy reaches deeply into, and corrects, the energies of life that animate our bodies and our minds.

TAKING HOMEOPATHIC REMEDIES WITH ORTHODOX MEDICINES

The question is often asked 'Do I have to stop taking my ordinary medicine when I start homeopathy?' Usually the answer is 'No'. Both the medicines will work normally, unaffected by each other. The main exceptions are antibiotics and oral steroids; these usually prevent homeopathic remedies from working (see below and chapter 6.)

Case Study

This is a case where the patient continued to take a large number of orthodox medicines without affecting her homeopathic treatment.

The patient is a lady aged 75. She has pains in her arms due to arthritis of the neck. She has sinusitis: the pain and catarrh disturb her sleep. But her sleep is affected even more by her very painful and swollen knees which also hurt a lot at other times. She also has chronic bronchitis. She used to get angina and breathlessness; this is now controlled by medication. She takes the following medicines:

Becanase, a nasal spray; hypermellose drops for her eyes; Codyranol, a painkiller; Movelat, an anti-inflammatory drug; for her heart she takes beta-blockers, calcium-channel blockers, isosorbide dinitrate, a nitrolingual spray and diuretics.

Her homeopathic symptoms included a sensitivity to draughts and a worsening of many of her problems at 3am. Treatment with *kali carbonicum*, a potentization of the mineral potassium carbonate, gave her a great deal of relief. The sinusitis, bronchitis and arthritis were very much better for several months after each short course of homeopathic treatment. She continued to take the orthodox medication because she felt unsure about the dangers of reducing it.

Once the homeopathy is working then most orthodox medicines can be stopped. This should usually be done gradually so the body has time to adjust. With some medicines the dose must be reduced very gradually. In some cases it is not safe to reduce the orthodox medication at all or only under medical supervision. Some treatments for high blood pressure and heart conditions are in this category. If there is any doubt consult your doctor and homeopath.

Considerations such as these sometimes, but very rarely, make homeopathic treatment impossible. Each case must be assessed on its own merits; it is best to ask a homeopath for advice before making an appointment if you think this question may apply to you.

Apart from this, homeopathy is capable of working wonders for the health of all age groups in almost all kinds of illness. Many people telephone me to ask whether homeopathy can help the problem they have. Ninety-nine times out of a hundred the answer is 'Yes'.

WHAT HOMEOPATHY CAN DO FOR YOU

Homeopathy is a safe natural system of medicine which does not have side effects, although symptoms can sometimes get worse for a short time before they get better. The remedies are inexpensive, non-toxic and have a pleasant taste.

It is suitable for all age groups from newborn babies to the very old. It is excellent in pregnancy and childbirth.

There are examples above of treatment of the elderly and during pregnancy. The following example completes the range of ages.

Case Study (Homeopathic Treatment of a Baby)
This was one of the first babies I ever treated. He was ten weeks old, born three weeks prematurely and suffering from colic. He was arching his back and head backwards and crying with each attack of pain. The GP had diagnosed an intestinal blockage. Glycerin suppositories cleared this but the colic soon began again. He could go for up to five days without passing a stool. Shortly, the colic became very severe, his arms started to jerk as he fell asleep.

There are several homeopathic remedies to choose from for this kind of colic. Only one of them has in its proving jerking of the limbs on falling asleep. This remedy is *belladonna*, and it worked extremely well for this child. The cause of the trouble was probably spasm of the intestinal muscles, arising from underdevelopment of the bowel. This was corrected by the remedy so the problem was tackled at its source.

Homeopathic treatment can be beneficial for the whole range of human diseases.

1 Infectious diseases from sore throats and scabies to measles and pneumonia.
2 Diseases of all the major systems of the human body:
of the *heart and circulatory system*, from high blood pressure and heart conditions to varicose veins;
of the *respiratory system*, including croup and asthma;
of the *digestive system*, from mouth ulcers to colitis;
of the *urinary and reproductive systems of both men and women*, for example cystitis and kidney infections; and in women endometriosis and other gynaecological conditions, and in men enlarged prostate and impotence;
of the *hormonal and nervous systems*, including meningitis, multiple sclerosis, thyroid disorders and all kinds of period problems;
of the *skin*, for example eczema, psoriasis, acne, warts and verrucas;
of the *musculo-skeletal system*: the effectiveness of homeopathy in back problems is not often appreciated; it helps the body to adjust and align itself; apart from that it is very effective in sports injuries and all rheumatic and arthritic problems.
3 Being holistic, homeopathy treats the mind and the emotions as well:
mental problems: these may be minor, such as poor concentration in students, or failing memory, or conditions arising from serious pathology like Alzheimer's disease;
emotional problems: all kinds of emotional problems respond very well to homeopathy: insomnia, anxiety, panic attacks, phobias, obsessions, manic-depression, violent and aggressive behaviour; currently many parents are seeking homeopathic treatment for hyperactivity in children.
4 Homeopathy is a godsend in psychosomatic disorders, or for cases where it is not known whether there is a physical basis for the symptoms. Either way, the same treatment will be

required and the correct homeopathic remedy will work. This is because the remedy enables the vital energy of the patient to do whatever is necessary for healing, whether a mental or a physical change is needed.

Case Study

A woman aged 32 came to see me with a diagnosis of angina neurosis. She has had this for 18 months since her father died of a heart attack. She gets heart pain, worse at times of stress. She also has insomnia and premenstrual mood changes. I had treated her three times before over a period of five years for eczema, catarrhal problems and insomnia. Each time she had done very well on her constitutional remedy, *arsenicum album*. This remedy also sorted out her heart problem.

5 One of the main benefits of homeopathy has not been mentioned. This is simply *feeling better*. Feeling better in yourself is often the first sign of a remedy working. An all-round improvement follows.

Case Study

A man aged 30 came for treatment for throat, gum and teeth problems, with swelling of his lips and left cheek, which is changing his appearance. In addition he has psoriasis. His biggest problems, however, are lack of motivation and creativity (he is a freelance writer), and difficulties with his concentration and memory.

A month after taking his remedy, *lachesis*, his physical condition showed little change. However his wife said he was a transformed person; he had created a new business which proved to be very successful. The physical problems also got better.

Most of the diseases listed above need treatment from a homeopathic practitioner. Homeopathy can also be used for first aid and for minor illnesses in the home. Equipped with a first aid kit of basic remedies and an introductory book such as this, you can learn how to treat yourself and your family and friends. You will discover that the correct remedies work very quickly for these problems, and that they tend to improve your general level of health.

Understanding the Basics

Homeopathy offers a safe natural way of treating most health problems. If you are looking for an alternative to the treatments you are familiar with, homeopathy is well worth investigation. Many people come to homeopathy as a last resort, when they have not been able to find help elsewhere. Others first start using homeopathy as a preventative, before any serious illness develops. Often they have made an informed decision to follow natural methods as their first choice. They will use antibiotics or other orthodox treatments if their preferred choices fail. For them, orthodox treatments are the last resort. For some of us, this change in priorities comes when we become parents and want to give our children only natural medicines. We often feel even more committed for our children than for ourselves to using only natural methods of treatment.

2

Human Beings, Health and Disease

NOT EVERYONE CATCHES FLU

WHY IS IT THAT ONE person exposed to a flu epidemic will go down with it when another will not? Or perhaps you know someone who had a headache and felt tired for a day or two, while your bout of flu knocked you out for weeks.

There have been a number of cases of meningitis in Britain in the 1980s and 90s. Why can we all have the meningococcal bacteria in our throats but only a very few of us actually develop the disease? Why does it prove fatal for one person yet another receiving the same treatment recovers completely?

> There is an infection of the majority to be sure, but it is confined to the rhinopharynx and usually goes unnoticed by the infected people . . . The cases of meningitis are the exception. The rule for meningococcal infection is benign, transient infection of the upper respiratory tract, hardly an infection at all, more like an equable association. It is still a mystery that meningitis develops in some patients, but it is unlikely that this represents a special predilection of the bacteria; it may be that the defence mechanisms of affected patients are flawed in some special way, so that the meningococci are granted access, invited in, so to say.[3]

The severity of an infection does not depend only on the virulence of the bacteria; the ability of the immune system to combat the bacteria is important too. Professor Lewis Thomas' words echo the homeopathic view exactly. The most important cause of disease is the 'flawed defence mechanism'.

PREDISPOSITION TO DISEASE

Homeopaths call a flaw in the defence mechanism, or a constitutional weakness, a predisposition to disease. It is a tendency to, or an openness to, a certain kind of illness.

Case Study

I treated a two-year-old girl for eczema which began after she had chicken pox three weeks previously. Before that she had been very clingy, ever since her mother had been away for a week. She is a warm-blooded, shy girl who loves being outdoors. After a dose of *pulsatilla 30* she was herself again, and had no eczema.

This case shows how a constitutional sensitivity results in illness. For this patient the separation from her mother affected her deeply. It knocked her vital energy off its normal course. Compounded by the chicken pox, another influence which she was susceptible to and unable to recover from, the result was eczema. *Pulsatilla* types are especially sensitive to separation from loved ones. Their constitutions can also be unduly affected by childhood illnesses. The gaps in our defences are our *predispositions*.

Predispositions are built into our constitutions by our inheritance and are influenced by environmental factors during our lives. Susceptibility to disease is a question of both nature and nurture. Predispositions can be triggered into actual illness by allergens, infection, stress, emotional and physical trauma, by bad diet and lifestyle, by aging and the developmental stages of life such as teething, puberty and menopause, and by many other factors.

The main cause of all disease is predisposition to it. Our predispositions determine what diseases we get and how badly they affect us.

Here is another example of how predispositions work. Even in two cases of the same disease the predispositions are not the same:

Case Studies – Asthma

The first is a 14-year-old boy who has had asthma, hay fever and eczema since he was a baby. He uses Becotide and Ventolin and cortisone creams regularly. He used a nebulizer for several years. The asthma prevents him from doing sports, and he gets depressed about always having to take one medicine or another. His hands itch, crack and bleed. When he is very wheezy his face sweats profusely.

He is a loner, with a tendency to go quiet when upset. He is sensitive to criticism and personal comments. If he is very low he can be tearful, when with his mother or on his own. Both the eczema and the asthma are much better when he is at the seaside.

The remedy *natrum muriaticum*, repeated several times over the next few years, kept this young man free of asthma, eczema and hay fever for the whole of that time.

The second case is of a little girl aged one year who has been diagnosed as asthmatic. There is a family history of asthma and allergies. From birth she had eczema; at three months it got better after cortisone cream was applied. Since four months she has had severe attacks of coughing and can become dehydrated and exhausted with them. She has been hospitalized. There is some damage to her lungs which is healing. The cough is dry while her breathing is bubbly.

She eats only small amounts and is underweight. She has had several ear infections and has needed antibiotics.

The only foods she is at all interested in are sweet things, puréed apple and fromage frais. She can get cross and refuse food. She cries if she is touched by anyone other than her family.

Her remedy was *antimonium tartaricum*. After the first dose she got a skin eruption on her scalp and her condition improved in every way. Six doses over the next four years kept her in very good health – thriving and free of illness.

This shows how individual our illnesses are. If we study each person and their illness carefully, we find that no two cases are identical. Homeopaths are very interested in these individual patterns. Every change in health and every symptom of illness maps out for us the constitution of the sick person. Paracelsus wrote, 'All diseases originate in the constitution. It is necessary that the constitution be known in order to know the disease.'

In the two cases above, the only similarity is the diagnosis of asthma; the actual state of health of the two cases is very different. The asthma is the tip of the iceberg. Treatment with inhalers will give only temporary relief by suppressing the end product of the disease state. This may be life-saving at times but to cure the asthma the whole system must be reorganized.

Disease is a condition not a thing. To compare ourselves with motor vehicles for a moment, remember that there is nothing called brake failure which our cars can catch. No virus attacks brake linings (except in science fiction). Brake failure is simply brakes failing to work. Similarly arthritis does not exist apart from the arthritic joints of patients. Arthritis is not an evil entity ready to attack us.

THE ENERGY OF LIFE: VITAL ENERGY

Every seven years our entire physical body is replaced. After seven years not a single molecule remains of the previous body. This includes the DNA molecules. Yet no one would deny that we are the same human being. Clearly the continuity does not come from the physical substance. The continuity is provided by an organizing principle, a formative energy which controls and maintains the human body. This formative energy is at work every moment energizing the processes of life. It is the form for the ever-changing physical content. For example, it guides the transformation of our food into our bodily structure. Besides the daily miracle of turning our breakfast into bone tissue, this blueprint of human individuality keeps all the systems of the human body working in harmony together. When we remember that a full understanding of even one of these systems is beyond us, then the enormity of this achievement in every moment becomes clear. The maintenance of this human form and the maintenance of health are one and the same process. Illness occurs if this process breaks down. Disease starts as a disorder of life energy, not of physical substance.

Case Study

At 3pm one afternoon a mother came in to my clinic to ask for help for her 17-year-old daughter. She has a bad throat infection with a high temperature. She is getting weak and dehydrated.

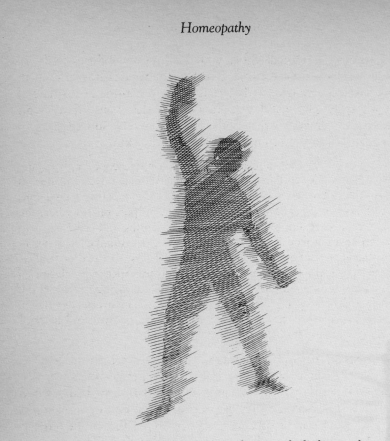

Figure 2   Vital energy permeates and surrounds the human form.

The patient herself has a baby daughter and the supply of breast milk is diminishing leading to problems for the baby. The following information reveals the homeopathic remedy required: she has a metallic taste in her mouth and is talking quickly and faintly.

One hour after one dose of *mercury 200* the patient's mother phoned me. There was no change in the illness at all. However the patient was 'a different person'. She was herself again and her energy was back. Over that evening the infection disappeared and the patient was very well by the following day.

The energy released into the system by the homeopathic medicine first appeared in the patient being better in herself. Then, guided by the organism's innate intelligence, it moved on to strengthen the weak point – her immune system.

A person is a unified whole with healing capabilities built in. These just need activating. The role of *vital energy* is crucial. The awesome magic of the human body cannot be explained on a purely physical level. Supporting this view, here is an American surgeon writing about a relatively simple part of ourselves that we often take for granted, the skin.

> Gaze upon the skin as I have, through a microscope brightly, and tremble at the wisdom of God, for here is a magic tissue to suit all seasons. Two layers compose the skin – the superficial epidermis and, deeper, the dermis. Between is a plane of pure energy where the life-force is in full gallop. Identical cells spring full-grown . . . to form an unbroken line over the body . . . this number marches in well-stepped soldiery, gallantly summoned to a sacrifice beyond its ken . . . let the skin be cut or burned, and the brigade breaks into a charge, fanning out laterally across the wound, racing to seal off the defect. The margins are shored up; healing earthworks are raised, and guerrilla squads of invading bacteria are isolated and mopped up. Hurrah for stratified squamous epithelium![4]

'. . . a plane of pure energy where the life-force is in full gallop': this is the source of health. This energy permeates the whole body and maintains health – unless it is functioning badly, when disease is the result. In the case of the skin diseases, for example, the real cause is a disturbance in the ability of the vital energy to maintain the process of producing healthy skin. This piece of writing conveys very effectively how health and disease are one process and that disease is a result of malfunctioning life energy.

Case Study
This is the case of a young woman of 22. Her psoriasis had been called by her skin specialist the worst case in the county. It began when she was three years old. The patches of affected skin were very widespread. Homeopathically she is a *pulsatilla* type. Improvement began a few days after taking the remedy, and three months later the psoriasis was 80 per cent better. At the time of writing it is still improving. She is also calmer and stronger in herself.

THE ENERGY THAT KEEPS US ALIVE IS THE ENERGY THAT KEEPS US HEALTHY

This *vital energy*, which is a central principle of homeopathy, has many names. Hippocrates called it 'the healing force of nature', alchemists called it 'vital fluid'. In acupuncture it is *chi*, in yoga *prana*. Like magnetism and electricity and all forms of energy, it cannot be seen but is clearly detectable by its effects.

> What does occur at the moment of death? The organism is structurally intact, cells are busily functioning, chemical reactions are still proceeding, yet a sudden change occurs and the body begins to decompose! Reflection upon this fact renders the concept of vital forces not only understandable, but appealing.[5]

The life force which departs at death is the difference between living tissue and dead tissue. It inhabits and animates our living bodies, protecting living tissue from disintegration and decay. It is like the magnet behind the paper which draws the iron filings into patterns.

To illustrate this, consider just one of the millions of self-regulating and self-healing activities which our bodies perform. If an infection develops in a wound then the immune system springs into action. Inflammation brings white blood cells to the wound to eliminate the invaders. These cells are transported via the circulatory system from the bone marrow. The 'intelligence system' of the body may cause the hypothalamus to adjust its thermostat to produce a high temperature. This accelerates body activity generally and increases antibody production.

One simple self-regulating activity can involve many body systems. Our self-healing systems are part of our anatomy and physiology. The normal processes of life and the maintenance of health are totally integrated.

Vital energy invisibly permeates our physical bodies, working without our conscious involvement. It is creative, formative and intelligent. Homeopaths believe that it is responsible for the state of our health. In health this vibrant energy is strong and harmonious. When this energy is weak or out of balance, we become ill. In other words, if our health breaks down it is because our vital energy has failed, allowing disorder to creep in where the harmonious forces of life are not in control. Health is life energy benevolently controlling its physical bodily realm.

Strong vital energy enables us and our bodies to bounce back to health when we come up against things that can trigger disease. The 'inflatable castles' that our children enjoy always have leaks, but as long as the motor is powerful, the castle will retain its bounce. Good vital energy is like that motor: it compensates for the inevitable daily demands on our bodies and minds and gives us some bounce to spare. Without this vitality disease can move into the vacuum and take over. In disease the motor is failing. The vital energy needs to be enhanced, unblocked, strengthened, harmonized, or one could almost say, re-educated or reprogrammed.

SCIENTIFIC CONFIRMATION OF VITAL ENERGY

1 **Kirlian Photography** This is a special technique of photography which shows that all objects, living or non-living, are surrounded by energy fields. Bright patterns are seen around a healthy person. When the person is ill the Kirlian photographs become weaker and more chaotic.
2 **Relativity** The most famous equation in science is Einstein's $E=mc^2$. This small but highly important equation states that energy and matter can be interchangeable. This has been confirmed by experiment. So the physical matter of our bodies is not the fixed foundation of our existence; we must concede a role to energy in our understanding of substance and therefore of disease.
3 **New Physics** Physicists now take this further. In order to explain the subatomic world they have been forced to conclude that another unknown level of reality exists. The subatomic particles of physical matter are constantly appearing out of, and disappearing back into, this other level of existence. The old theories of solid substance have dematerialized between our fingers. All things, including human beings, are the unfolded parts of a quantum sea of potential existence. So our physical bodies depend for their existence upon an invisible backcloth of potentiality. There is a similar relationship between health and vital energy. Vital energy is the invisible backcloth which determines our health.
4 **The Memory Of Water** Research by the famous French immunologist Jacques Benveniste, published in the scientific

31

journal *Nature*, has shown that homeopathic remedies leave an energy pattern in the water used to dilute them. In effect, water has a memory. Another intriguing example of this is found in snowflakes. All snowflakes have their own unique crystal structure, despite their astronomical numbers. Yet melted snowflakes have been frozen again and have resumed the same original crystal shape.

It is not the substance that is producing these effects, but the formative force or pattern of energy it carries. Like human organisms, homeopathic remedies possess vital energy. When the remedy is taken this energy is transmitted to the patient.

THE HOLISTIC VIEW OF HEALTH

Body and mind are a continuum. They cannot be separated and they influence each other. The sight of a lion produces adrenalin, the thought of a good meal produces digestive enzymes. Consciousness and substance are indivisibly linked in a living human organism. The psychologist C G Jung describes how the lower regions of the mind blend into the physical body:

> The deep 'layers' of the psyche lose their individual uniqueness as they retreat further and further into darkness. 'Lower down', that is to say as they approach the autonomous functional systems, they . . . are : . . extinguished in the body's materiality, i.e. in chemical substance.[6]

We must regard a human being as a unified mind-body system. The health of the mind or the body is dependent on the health of the whole. A sickness of part of the human being is a sickness of the whole.

This is the philosophy of *holism* applied to health and disease; the whole is greater than the sum of the parts. The essence of a human being cannot be found in any one part, not in body, mind, cell, or gene, nor indeed in all the parts together. It is something more than all the constituent parts. Plato, the Ancient Greek philosopher, said: 'The cure of the part should not be attempted without treatment of the whole. No attempt should be made to cure the body without the soul, and if the head and body are to be healthy you must begin by curing the mind.' D H Lawrence supports this view in his poem *Healing*:

I am not a mechanism, an assembly of various sections,
And it is not because the mechanism is working wrongly that I am
ill.[7]

We see holograms in science exhibitions and on credit cards. One of the extraordinary things about them is that the whole image can be re-created from a small part of it. If the part is too small the image may be fuzzy, but it is still complete. This gives us a graphic example of how holism works. The whole transcends the parts. There is a law in cybernetics which states that for any organized system there will be a higher level from which the organization comes.

SELF-HEALING SYSTEMS AND SELF-HELP

Our integral self-healing systems provide adjustments and responses to constant changes in our environments and our lives. The responses are unified through many systems and levels of organization. The body processes include constant electrical, chemical and physical activity. The level of intelligence involved is awe-inspiring.

Homeopathy is one way of strengthening your system and helping to achieve a natural balance emotionally and physically. Emotional stress directly affects the physical body. The reverse also holds: our psychological state is affected by our bodies, thus the whole system becomes stronger when homeopathic treatment works.

We can also assist our vital energy in keeping us healthy by finding the problems in our lives which are draining it. Conflicts in relationships, frustrations at work, negative emotions, damaging patterns of behaviour can all consume our precious vitality so that there is less available to maintain good health. Then our predispositions are uncovered and illness develops. By giving positive attention to all aspects of our lives and finding ways of working through the problems we put less strain on ourselves.

If you are at ease with yourself this will help to keep your body free of 'dis-ease'. This gives us two meanings for the word 'disease'. 'Dis-ease' is being out of balance in mind and body; the harmony of the whole organism is disturbed. A state of dis-ease leads to the increased possibility of disease in the usual sense of the word.

Whatever constitution you have, weak or strong, you can make the best of your endowment by healthy living. This means eating fresh natural foods, organic if possible, and not burdening your body too much with tobacco and alcohol etc, even if you have a constitution that can cope with it.

We tend to resort to these props when we are under stress, and stress cannot necessarily be avoided. Looking after your emotional health is therefore very important because you will not be reaching for the cigarettes, whisky, extra food or tranquillizers if you are at ease with yourself.

Case Study

A woman aged 49 wanted help with migraines and menopausal problems which have recently got worse. With the migraines she has lots of vomiting and has to lie in a darkened room for 24 hours. Hormone replacement therapy helped the hot flushes but made the migraines worse so she stopped taking it.

She went on to describe the background to these problems. She is divorced and the relationship with her ex-husband is stressful. Since he left she has been on automatic pilot. She tends to chew over problems, sleep badly and lose her temper, though recently she controls this. The homeopathic picture is filled out by the following: she likes order, is methodical and gets impatient if people do not do what they say they will.

The migraines and menopausal problems have been thrown up by a system under stress. This lady is not at ease with herself or her life and her health is suffering as a result. Twenty-four hours after taking *nux vomica* she had an unexpected migraine with lots of hot flushes. Then she had no more of either problem for five months. She told me that she was now able to speak to her ex-husband about their son without losing her temper. A relapse after five months was caused by drinking coffee. A repeat dose of *nux vomica* put things right again. She needed another dose three months later and has been fine since then.

HOMEOPATHY: HOLISTIC NATURAL MEDICINE

When we understand ourselves in the way described here then we will prefer treatments which respect our bodies as self-healing systems. We are intricate and beautiful beings; medicines can work with the natural forces which maintain our health. Medicines should also respect our individual patterns of illness. They should go to the core of the problem, which is in the core of ourselves. The whole, which is something more than all the parts, must be healed. Homeopathy is one of the medical systems which can give these benefits. The next chapter explains how it works.

3

How Homeopathy Works

HOMEOPATHY WORKS BECAUSE its two main pillars, *the law of similarity* and *potentization*, complement each other. Together they make up the homeopathic system – a system of medicine which can make a tremendous contribution to health care. Before this can happen patients and medical practitioners need a better understanding of how homeopathy works. The explanation in this chapter starts with a look at how orthodox medicines work and this, in turn, highlights the different approach taken in homeopathic medicine. The chapter goes on to explore this approach and the mechanism of action of the medicines. Ideas from modern science which help us to understand homeopathy are included.

THE ALLOPATHIC AND HOMEOPATHIC APPROACHES

When we take an anti-inflammatory drug for an arthritic hip its effect is to alter the biochemistry of the body. The presence of medicine neutralizes the inflammation. The hip will therefore feel better. When we take a sleeping tablet we are swallowing chemicals that induce sleep. The active ingredient enters our internal chemical laboratory and, until it is dispersed, corrects the imbalance that is causing sleeplessness. In both these examples the medication can be repeated as necessary to maintain the right biochemical levels.

Homeopaths have some questions at this point. Why is there

this inappropriate inflammation of the hip in the first place? It is not only unnecessary, because there is no injury to repair or foreign body to expel, it is positively harmful. The body is making a mistake – it is malfunctioning. Part of its organization has broken down.

The cause of the disease is not in the hip, nor even in the inflammatory process, which is an essential part of the defence mechanism. The cause is in the self-regulating system which initiates the misplaced inflammation. In the case of sleeplessness, the cause is that the patient's metabolism is stuck in waking mode.

In the allopathic medical treatment described above, the problem is being relieved temporarily by each dose of medication. The body all along is still trying to produce the inflammation. Homeopaths suggest the possibility of assisting the body's own self-regulation. Instead of targeting the end product of the malfunction, would it be possible to correct the process at its source? Could a medicine correct the body's regulatory system so that it no longer produces the inflammation? Could a medicine be given for sleeplessness that will enable the body to sleep naturally?

This medicine would act on the self-regulating systems of the body rather than directly on the physical level. It would reprogramme this system to bring it back to a normal healthy pattern. In effect, it would point out to the body its mistake. It would treat the body as an intelligent self-governing organization.

WHY HOMEOPATHIC MEDICINE MUST BE SIMILAR TO THE DISEASE

Homeopaths suggest that this vital regulatory system can work properly if it is given the right stimulus. And the right stimulus is a mimic of the disease which then produces a healing response from the vital energy. We tend to underestimate the wisdom of the body. Most illnesses are healed without any medicine at all. When they are not, then the vital energy only needs the right encouragement. Homeopathic remedies work with the natural efforts of the body, guiding them in the right direction.

This is why the medicine given in homeopathic treatment is similar to the disease. The homeopathic remedy acts as a version of the disorder that the human organism responds to. The response will be the reorganization that is needed to re-establish health. The organism's innate healing intelligence will do whatever is necessary.

The law of similarity works by drawing a response from the body's own healing abilities. The homeopathic remedy produces a reaction from the creative life energy hidden within each of us.

Example: The Homeopathic Remedy Coffea tosta *For Insomnia*
You have a cup of coffee when you need to be alert and motivated, quick-thinking and resourceful. A material dose of *coffea tosta*, an infusion of ground roast coffee beans, can produce that state for you. But what should you do if you are in that state and do not want to be? Perhaps you have been to a very intense meeting or a very exciting party one evening and afterwards cannot get to sleep. Or something really good has happened in your life and your mind is full of ideas and your body is restless. In these circumstances a homeopathic dose of *coffea tosta* will neutralize this state and bring peace and rest. A material dose induces that state, a homeopathic dose neutralizes it by evoking a response from your vital energy.

EXAMPLES OF 'LIKE CURES LIKE' IN SCIENCE AND EVERYDAY LIFE

The law of similarity can be found outside the world of homeopathy. Here are examples from science, literature and other fields. Some are included to support the theory of homeopathy rather than give watertight proof of its validity. They show the power similar things have over each other. Like can cure like. Also similar things have the power to attract, repel, enhance and inhibit each other, depending on the circumstances.

1 The first known statement of the law of similarity in medical writing was made by Hippocrates (who is the origin of the Hippocratic Oath, and is widely accepted as the father of Western medicine.): 'Through the like, disease is produced, and through the application of the like, disease is cured.'
2 Paracelsus echoed Hippocrates when he wrote: 'Arsenic cures disease due to an exaltation of the arsenical quality in man.

What corresponds to brain in the outside world cures disease of the human brain, and so on.'

3 In science the *law of interference* states that waves of the same frequency but from different sources will neutralize each other. In homeopathy the disease and the remedy are of the same frequency but from different sources. The remedy comes from a naturally occurring substance, the disease comes from the patient. When the two meet they eliminate each other.

4 Resonance occurs when two things vibrate at a similar rate. If you play the middle C of one piano, then the middle C of a piano nearby will sound in sympathy. This shows the power there is in similarity.

5 A modern theory of evolution proposed by biologist Rupert Sheldrake suggests that each species of living thing has its own life energy. This affects every member of that species by means of the resonance between them. To illustrate this idea Sheldrake points out that when a new synthetic chemical is made for the second time, it forms much more quickly and easily than it did the first time, even on the other side of the world. This phenomenon has been confirmed frequently by experiment.

6 The law of similars is occasionally applied unwittingly in orthodox medicine in desensitization treatments and in immunizations. (In both these cases it is used without the other principles of homeopathy.) Incidentally, Edward Jenner developed his smallpox vaccination in the same year that Samuel Hahnemann published his first work on homeopathy.

7 Empathy is crucial in the relationship between any practitioner and patient. Empathy is based on being able to share in another's suffering by knowing something of that suffering oneself. Often the best counsellors for, say, victims of abuse are people who have themselves experienced abuse. The pain in the therapist is curative of the similar pain in the client.

8 In psychotherapy it is acknowledged that to heal a traumatic experience it is necessary to re-experience the pain. In the safety of the therapy a suffering which is similar to the original suffering can be endured, and thereby healed.

9 In Greek mythology one of the great healers is Chiron. He had an incurable wound. This gave him his healing role and is the origin of the idea of the 'wounded healer'. Through their own suffering healers know how to heal the suffering of their patients.

10 Shakespeare writes in *Romeo and Juliet*:

> Tut man, one fire burns out another's burning;
> One's pain is lessened by another's anguish,
> Turn giddy and be helped by backward turning
> One desperate grief cures with another's languish.
> Take thou some new infection to the eye,
> And the rank poison of the old will die.

11 The Oracle at Delphi said: 'That which makes sick shall heal.'

These examples are all based on the law of similarity: 'like influences, responds to, and cures, like.' Homeopathy is one very powerful demonstration of this law.

POTENTIZATION

Potentizing a medicine is not only a method of diluting it to reduce side effects. It achieves much more than this. Paradoxically, the process also *increases* the strength of the medicine for a person who needs it. For the person whose health problems correspond to that medicine, one dose will have a powerful beneficial effect. For others for whom it is not the right remedy, many doses will do nothing. The remedy *phosphorus* cured a patient of nosebleeds. A relative who suffered from the same problem treated himself for several weeks with a whole bottle of *phosphorus* tablets. This had no effect on him at all. It is the quality of similarity which triggers the therapeutic effect, not the quantity of doses.

Potentization of a medicine gives it special properties. The therapeutic effect is increased while the toxic effect is reduced.

As the remedies are serially diluted they are also *succussed*, that is, they are shaken in a predetermined way a set number of times. On the most commonly used scale of potencies, the medicine is diluted one part in 100, then shaken 50 times. The process is repeated five times more to produce the sixth potency on the centesimal scale, 6c. This is a low potency. Repetition of the dilution 30 times yields the 30th potency, which is still quite low. The 200th, 1,000th and 10,000th potencies are high potencies.

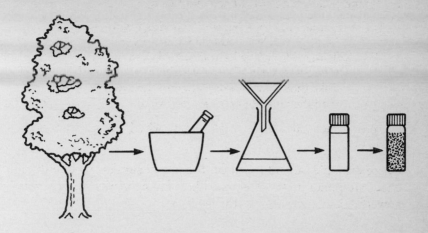

Figure 3   Making a homeopathic remedy. A sample of the substance is pulverized, mixed with alchohol, filtered and then potentized. The resulting liquid is used to medicate tablets.

Preparation of a Homeopathic Remedy: Silica

I have chosen *silica* as an example because it shows how even an insoluble substance is turned into a homeopathic remedy. The starting point is flint, one of the many natural forms of *silicon dioxide*. This is ground into a powder, then ground in a mortar and pestle with lactose for three hours. After that it can be potentized in the same way as a soluble substance. One part of this preparation is mixed with 99 parts of alcohol and succussed. Each repetition of this process raises the potency one step higher.

The amount of the original substance in homeopathic medicines is unbelievably small. This apparently straightforward method takes us through the physical structure of the substance into its underlying energy field. We know beyond doubt from modern physics that the particles which make up physical matter are 'concentrations of energy which come and go'[8]. The particles appear briefly out of a sea of quantum energy and soon disappear back into it. Matter is merely the visible part of an energy field. This is not over-enthusiastic wishful thinking but demonstrable fact. Given the right conditions, science has shown that matter and energy are interchangeable. Potentization is a method of making the energy available which is hidden in matter.

For example the *silica* sample above could provide enough high potency tablets to treat thousands of people. With remedies made from animals, in most cases a product such as milk or blood or venom from an animal is used. In a very few instances the life of an animal has been taken. One life is enough simply because the remedies are so dilute. For example the remedy *tarentula* was made from a spider killed 100 years ago. Even now all preparations of this remedy originate from that one spider.

EXAMPLES OF THE EFFECTIVENESS OF VERY HIGH DILUTIONS

1 In biology the Arndt-Schultz law states that very strong stimuli are harmful to living organisms whereas very small ones are beneficial. Small stimuli activate our responses.
2 There are many instances of animals being affected by extremely small concentrations of hormones, enzymes and other substances. For example, insects are attracted by pheromones from the opposite sex at huge distances. In the sea sharks can detect extraordinarily small amounts of blood.
3 Inside the human body concentrations of thyroid hormone of one part in 10,000 parts of blood lead to marked changes in metabolic processes.
4 The human sense of smell can detect the substance mercaptan when there is only one part present in 500,000,000,000 parts of air.

The appendix gives a selection of all the laboratory tests which have been done on the effects of homeopathic potencies on enzymes, blood antibodies, plant growth rates etc. The scientific evidence shows that the potencies have definite effects.

CONCLUSION

Chaos theory and complexity theory have shown that we can revolutionize our understanding of how the universe works. Can we take this revolution far enough to make homeopathy scientifically acceptable?

Science is closer than we might think to providing an explanation for homeopathy. The parallels between long-established homeopathic principles and recent scientific discoveries are gratifying for homeopaths and open up exciting possibilities for research.

There is a well-known example which illustrates chaos theory. The flap of a butterfly's wing in Australia can lead, via a long chain of increasing results, to a tornado in America. When a system is on the point of changing it takes very little to push it over the brink. A tiny change can trigger a gigantic change in a charged system but the small push must be in the direction the system is trying to go. This is how a very small dose of a medicine similar to the disease can bring about healing.

Case Study

This patient is a little boy of 18 months. He is very unhappy a lot of the time because of an emotional hypersensitivity. He cries and cries, and cannot stop, when looked at, touched, or approached, even by his parents. He does not want to be cuddled. When extremely upset he runs around the room hitting everything and moaning. He seems to resent help when in a bad mood – he pushes you away, yet cries more when left.

A well-known remedy for difficult children is *chamomilla*, but really impossible children who have this pattern of behaviour need the remedy *cina*. They put great stress on their parents because whatever you do for them makes them worse. At the follow-up visit six weeks later his mother described how he suddenly got worse as they were leaving the clinic. *The usual behaviour pattern was very intense for one hour and since then he has been a different child. The remedy gave him an extra push in the direction of healing.* Now he is cuddly, more courageous and assertive, and is no longer so sensitive.

Physicist David Bohm writes: 'Matter as we know it is a small "quantised" wave-like excitation on top of this background [of energy]. Further developments in physics may make it possible to probe the above mentioned background in a more direct way.'[9] Perhaps potentization is a method of probing which releases from matter its medical powers.

The most exciting thing about the many scientific revelations of recent years is the increased reverence for nature that scientists are developing. After four billion years of research and development, nature has produced solutions to countless problems whose existence has not even occurred to us. In this new atmosphere of wonderment rather than arrogance, homeopathy becomes more credible. Our bodies have subtleties and complexities we know nothing about. Many processes of life are beyond our understanding. Homeopathic medicines give us a means of healing which respects and enhances this creation which is beyond our understanding.

4

Your Visit to a Homeopath

HOW TO FIND AND CHOOSE A HOMEOPATH

CHOOSING WHO TO go to with your health problems should be a careful and informed decision. Perhaps it would be a good idea to make enquiries about several homeopaths who live near you. Here are some considerations to bear in mind.

1 *Qualifications*: You may want to check the homeopath's qualifications by speaking to them personally, or by contacting the relevant professional body (see chapter 1 and *Useful Addresses*).
2 *Reputation*: Take into account reports you have heard in your area, bearing in mind that no-one is going to be able to cure every case.
3 *Professionalism*: Your homeopath should have a professional way of working which will include the following: a suitable place of work, an organized appointments system, reasonable accessibility for enquiries and emergencies, proper storage for remedies and case files, assurance of confidentiality, and a commitment to the work of healing.
4 *Your homeopath should be someone you can get on with and in whom you have confidence*: Do you want to see a man or a woman? Do you want to meet the homeopath briefly and find out if you feel comfortable with him or her before committing yourself? Do you want to check beforehand that your problems can be helped by homeopathy? You could telephone and ask any questions you may have. Many homeopaths will offer

a short introductory appointment either free or for a small charge.

THE CONSULTATION: BEING THE PATIENT

This may be a new experience for you and it helps to know what is involved before you start. The section in chapter 1 called 'What It Is Like To Have Homeopathic Treatment' tells you a little. The hour or more with the homeopath will be spent compiling a full profile of you and your illness from a homeopathic perspective. In theory this can be divided into three stages:

1 The first is where you describe your problems to the homeopath. The homeopath may well encourage you to say more and ask if there is anything else until you have mentioned everything you can think of. You should tell him or her about whatever is troubling you – emotional difficulties or anything that is not going well in your life, as well as physical complaints.

2 Then the homeopath will want more details of all your problems. You may be asked direct and specific questions at this stage. You may be asked how and when each problem started and developed, what triggers or influences each symptom, how each pain feels, and so on.

3 The third stage is where the homeopath finds out more about you by asking the characteristic homeopathic questions: What foods do you strongly like or dislike? How are you affected by the seasons and different weather conditions? How well do you sleep? What are you afraid of? When do you get nervous? What do you worry about? How sociable are you? What experiences have had a deep effect on you? The answers give the homeopath an impression of your personality type and your outlook on life. However, don't stick strictly to the questions; use them as springboards to help you talk about yourself. Sometimes patients will tell homeopaths things they have never told anyone else. Be honest and open: this will help the homeopath find the right remedy for you and thus heal your illness.

You may start to think, that the homeopath believes your illness to be psychosomatic. This is not so, but homeopaths have found

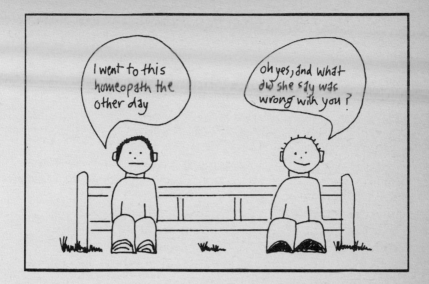

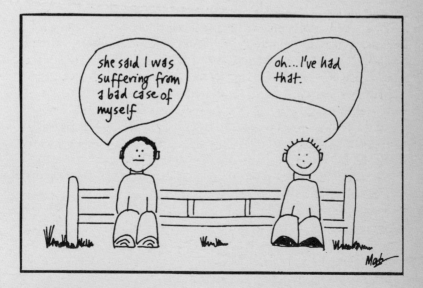

Figure 4   Reprinted by kind permission of John Boulderstone from "So You've Seen A Homeopath" by John and Katherine Boulderstone. Drawn by Martin Hobson, Helios Clinic, Tunbridge Wells, 1995.

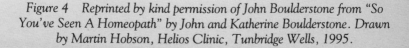

that a person's state of mind is a trustworthy guide to the remedy that will heal both body and mind.

The homeopath will be scrutinizing you carefully, but not being judgmental; his aim is to understand you as an individual. Information such as the diagnosis, test results, medical history, and the treatment you are already receiving is needed by the homeopath. But this is not important in the choice of remedy, so it is not the main concern of the consultation. Homeopaths are like detectives tracking down clues; they do not want to miss one, as that one clue could be the key to the whole case.

It is not easy for the patient to understand what the homeopath needs to know. Patients get concerned that they are giving the wrong kind of information with too much detail – or not enough. Here are some guidelines:

1 Try and simply supply information, for instance the time of day when you feel a certain pain or state of mind, rather than why you should experience it at that particular time. Noticing that eating cheese stops you sleeping is important; telling the homeopath that when you cannot sleep you start to fear that you have cancer is important too. Nothing more is needed; the homeopath does not interpret or explain such observations but just takes note of them.

2 Use your own words, not technical terms. Your own words give the homeopath a better impression of your personal experience of the problems.

3 Tell the truth about yourself, including your difficult side, like having a bad temper or being intolerant of certain things. The homeopath needs to know anything you are sensitive to. It may be helpful to mention the comments other people make about you.

Your deepest fears and secrets are very important in the choice of remedy. These things are not silly or shameful. The homeopath will have listened to such sensitive issues many times before, and mentioning them will be a great help.

Some people enjoy unburdening themselves in this way. For others it may be an invasion of personal space or a difficult confession. Homeopaths acknowledge that some issues may be too painful to uncover and will respect your wishes.

Equally, do not feel put off if you have no deep inner struggles: there will still be other things to talk about.

THE CONSULTATION: THE HOMEOPATH'S ROLE

The homeopath's first role is 'active listening'. This involves helping the patient to give the information that is needed. Patients may at times need gentle encouragement to express themselves. The aim is a complete case – a well-rounded 'portrait in words' of the patient.

During this process you may be able to sense the homeopath's mind working, absorbing the information you are giving and putting it into some kind of order. For the homeopath, each case is a jigsaw puzzle that can be assembled in many ways. He or she will try one way and get a picture that resembles, perhaps, the remedy *pulsatilla*. Putting the symptoms into a different pattern may produce a better likeness of the remedy *staphysagria*. Then a certain feature of the case may reveal a striking image of the remedy *cuprum*. Insight, knowledge of materia medica and homeopathic skills are working together here on the main challenge faced in homeopathy.

Each case is unique. The homeopath is reading the symptoms of the patient. Each symptom and characteristic of the person is a clue in this detective work. When the homeopath has enough clues he or she can understand the pattern lying behind the physical and psychological state and categorize each person as one of a hundred or more homeopathic types. You may then have to wait a few days before the homeopath has finished working out the remedy you need.

Case Study

This patient has severe panic attacks; the type of attack is very characteristic of a certain homeopathic remedy.

If she hears a plane flying overhead at night she fears that it will fall out of the sky on top of her. She listens for noises and cannot sleep. If a plane does go over, her heart will race and she will be awake for an hour. She is often afraid that something horrendous will happen; for instance, that on the way to work the bus will not be able to stop at the bottom of a hill. She is apprehensive generally; before something is going to happen she thinks about everything that could possibly go wrong and feels better once the event has taken place.

Such panic attacks are extremely debilitating and this lady

was having increasing problems carrying on her normal life. After the remedy *argentum nitricum*, potency 1m, these attacks disappeared completely and one year later she is still well.

ASSESSING THE TREATMENT

After taking the medicine according to the instructions, several weeks will elapse before your next appointment. During that time you should continue to avoid anything which might antidote the treatment. If the treatment is going well you will start to understand the homeopathic healing process. This has its own logic and sequence. If you have any questions telephone the homeopath.

The cure proceeds from within the body outwards and may take some time to reach the main problems. Very often patients will say 'I felt better in myself quite quickly. My main problem is not much better really, but I am coping with it and it is not affecting my life so much. It was worse for a couple of days at first.'

This is an excellent reaction to the treatment and must be allowed to unfold without interference. You can now feel confident that your illness is being cured at a deep level and you will soon experience a long period of much improved health.

Case Study

A lady of 31 came because of her eczema which she has had since she was three. There are patches all over her and it has been worse since her first pregnancy. During the pregnancy she felt the loss of her parents a few years previously. Her mother died of caner and her father died in a road accident. She describes herself as a 'sad soul' and says she has not cried for them. During the treatment the eczema got worse then she started to feel surprisingly well in herself despite having great difficulties with her skin. She was no longer getting upset about her parents. Over the next few weeks her skin improved steadily and later she was almost completely better.

At the second visit you should report all the changes you have noticed. Keeping notes can be helpful but once a week is enough to record the overall trends. You will be asked about all the problems you mentioned in the first consultation so that the process of cure can be mapped. Sometimes, gradual changes only become apparent at this stage and after the follow-up consultation you realize how much has changed.

Patience is sometimes needed at this point. Some severe and long-standing conditions will get better very slowly and may have to get worse at first. Good homeopathic treatment can transform your health and your life but this may take some time. When the rewards are so great it is a shame to spoil the process and regret it later.

Patience will also be needed if the treatment is not working. The homeopath will then need to reconsider everything, and give you a new remedy.

THE CONSULTATION AS A LEARNING EXPERIENCE

Having homeopathic treatment can be a learning experience in several ways.

1 You may learn something about yourself or acknowledge new facets of yourself as a result of the consultation or the changes you feel after the treatment.
2 The in-depth interview and the stages of recovery are an education in the relationship of disease to human nature.
3 Above all, if you are intending to study homeopathy, then experiencing it personally is an unrivalled foundation for your developing knowledge. However, students of homeopathy and homeopaths themselves can sometimes be the worst patients because they see themselves in terms of all the different remedies. This affects how they describe themselves in the consultation.

Part II

Using
Homeopathy

5

Your Home Remedy Kit

WHICH REMEDIES TO GET FIRST

HOMEOPATHIC REMEDIES are becoming more easily available in health food stores and pharmacies. For a wider selection of remedies and potencies you can order from a specialist pharmacy (see *Useful Addresses*). Sets of remedies can be supplied in their own carrying cases. It is important to have a conventional first-aid kit and know conventional first-aid techniques, such as mouth to mouth resuscitation; this can be learned at a first-aid course. Keep a manual and bandages with your remedies and get a good family health handbook.

The introduction to homeopathy for many people is *arnica* which is often needed in accidents and injuries. It makes sense to start with *arnica* and expand your kit as funds allow.

The First-Aid Kit

The following remedies will cover most injuries and accidents including bites, stings and burns:

Arnica, bryonia, calendula, cantharis, hypericum, ledum, ruta and *rhus tox. Bellis perennis, symphytum, staphysagria* and *urtica* are needed less often and can be added if possible.

Calendula or *hypericulum/calendula* cream for cuts and grazes and a cream for minor burns would also be useful. Rescue Remedy or Five Flower Remedy, which are combinations of flower remedies introduced by Dr Edward Bach, are helpful in any shock or stress.

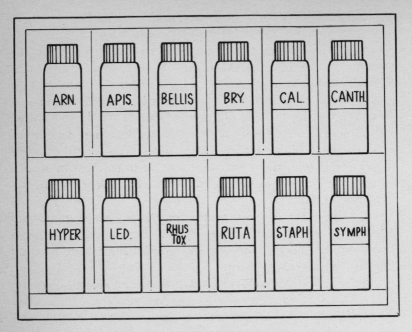

Figure 5 A homeopathic first-aid kit.

The Basic Home Remedy Kit

The next step is to build up a kit of the remedies most often needed for common illnesses:

Aconite, apis mellifica, arsenicum album, belladonna, chamomilla, ferrum phosphorica, gelsemium, ignatia, lachesis, lycopodium, mercury, nux vomica, phosphorus, pulsatilla, rhus tox., silica, sulphur, staphysagria.

The other remedies are used less often and can be added individually as needed.

STORING THE MEDICINES

Homeopathic remedies stored properly will last indefinitely. Open only the bottle you need, and for the shortest possible time. Do not put tablets back into the bottles once they have been taken out. Store your remedies in a cool dark place away from computer and TV screens and other electromagnetic fields.

HOW TO GIVE THE MEDICINES

Homeopathic tablets should never be touched, except by the patient just before they are taken. To take one, the patient should put it onto his or her clean hand or into something like a clean dry spoon, or into the cap of the remedy bottle, and put it straight into the mouth. The tablets should not be swallowed but allowed to dissolve under the tongue. This may take a few seconds or half an hour depending on the density of the tablet. The tablets are made of lactose – sugar of milk. Anyone who is lactose intolerant of even small quantities can take the remedies in liquid form.

For babies, if you cannot get the remedy as a liquid or as small granules, then a tablet can be crushed into a powder between two clean dry spoons. This way the baby will not be able to spit out the tablet or choke on it.

Giving remedies to animals sometimes requires ingenuity. Tablets crushed between two clean dry spoons into a powder can sometimes be put into the mouths of larger animals. For cats and dogs I usually dissolve several crushed tablets in a little milk or water. Otherwise follow the same procedures as for humans.

The time of day you take the tablet does not matter, but you must have nothing by mouth for half an hour before and after taking it – don't drink, eat, smoke, clean your teeth and so on. After a strong curry or other food with a persistent taste you may have to wait even longer for the taste to disperse. This time limit can be reduced to a few minutes if it is not possible to wait longer, especially if only water is being taken.

ANTIDOTES TO THE TREATMENT

While taking homeopathic treatment, and in the case of chronic illness for as long as the benefit continues, you should avoid having anything which stops the treatment working. Treatment for acute illness cannot be antidoted once the patient is better.

Some of the strongest antidotes are things containing camphor, eucalyptus and menthol. The damage is done by inhaling the vapour, so just smelling these things can antidote. Olbas oil, Vick, Carvol, Deep-Heat, and many other inhalants, muscle

1. Nothing by mouth for 20 minutes before taking a remedy.

2. Do not touch the tablet or powder

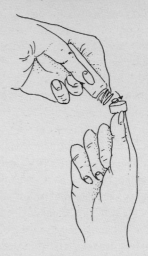

3. Taking the tablet.

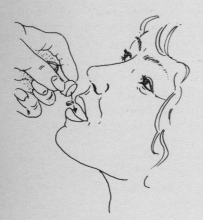

4. Allow the tablet to dissolve under your tongue and do not take anything else by mouth for 20 minutes.

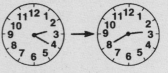

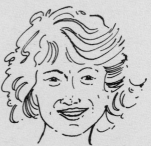

Figure 6   Taking a homeopathic remedy.

relaxants, lip salves and even mothballs must be strictly avoided. Recreational drugs also antidote homeopathy.

In addition, avoid drinking coffee. Even a few sips have been known to antidote on occasions. Weak instant decaffeinated coffee, and coffee cake or chocolates do not usually cause problems.

Most conventional medicines can be taken alongside homeopathic treatment – there will be no interference in either direction. (There may, however, be some confusion afterwards about which one has worked.) The exceptions to this are antibiotic tablets, steroid tablets, immunizations and anaesthetics of any kind, even local ones, and dental anaesthetics. If possible plan immunizations and dental work which requires an anaesthetic before, or at least two months after, homeopathic treatment for long-term problems. Once a patient has stopped taking antibiotic or steroid tablets homeopathic treatment can begin within two days. Remember that steroids and some other medicines can be discontinued only with medical supervision.

Be wary of treating anyone who is having, or has recently had, homeopathic treatment for long-term health problems. Giving any homeopathic remedies at this stage could interfere with the treatment. Contact the homeopath concerned first.

Emotional shocks and traumas can sometimes antidote the treatment. You may think you have antidoted your remedy, but a few days later you start to get better again. In treatment of chronic complaints it is important to wait for two weeks before repeating the remedy, to see if it really has been antidoted.

6

Before You Begin

THE STAGES OF HOMEOPATHIC TREATMENT

THERE ARE FIVE essential stages in all homeopathic treatment. This chapter explains these five stages to prepare you for applying the remedy pictures given later. The stages may seem rather obvious but remembering this sequence, especially during a health crisis, will help you to get the best out of homeopathy.

First you need to know some definitions. An *acute* illness is a short-term illness such as a cold, flu, pneumonia, appendicitis etc. It is something you normally recover from after a few days (or a few weeks with some of the severe ones). A *chronic* illness is one that tends to continue long-term and to get worse, such as eczema, irritable bowel syndrome and heart disease.

Acute illness can be *emergency*, *severe* or *mild*. With chronic illness this makes four categories. Each one will need different urgency of treatment, different assistance from the doctor, different dosage etc.

1 *Decide whether it is appropriate for you to give homeopathic treatment in this case* (The section 'How to use homeopathic remedies' on page 62 helps with this decision.)
2 *Take the case* Record all the information about the illness *and the patient*. This may range from one sentence such as 'I hit my finger with a hammer and it's gone blue and it hurts' to several pages of notes. Only when this is complete should you go on to step three.
3 *Analyse the case* To organize the case notes make a list of the

symptoms. From this you will be able to work out the remedy.

4 *Give the remedy* Decide which of the categories (from *emergency* to *chronic*) described in the tables on pages 62, 63 and 108 fits your case. Each category has its own guidance on dosage etc.

5 *Assess the reaction* Record the patient's reaction to the remedy and decide whether further treatment is needed. Keep all the records of each patient you treat as this helps with future treatment. (Sometimes subsequent illnesses will need the same remedy.)

Conducting a homeopathic consultation and selecting the remedy required are skills which develop with experience. You will know a little already if you have been to a homeopath or have read chapter 1 and chapter 4. If you also have the chance to observe a homeopath at work, do so. There is nothing better than live experience. Also try to practise on your friends. You can then study the notes and work out possible remedies without actually giving them, and learn a lot that way.

IS IT APPROPRIATE FOR YOU TO GIVE HOMEOPATHIC TREATMENT?

When you begin to use the remedies for yourself, family and friends, start with the conditions which are easiest to treat, such as minor injuries, and as you gain knowledge and confidence go on to more difficult problems. It is not unusual to have a period of beginner's luck at first, and then become over-enthusiastic, wanting to treat everyone and everything. Next comes a phase of disappointment when none of the remedies you give seem to work. This is an initiation into the enduring work of homeopathy and the dedication required to keep studying human nature and disease in the light of homeopathic knowledge. The next phase is one of maturity where you are less eager to show everyone that homeopathy can save the world, but are getting a consistent level of success. By now you will also be aware that you cannot rush up to every accident you see and give *arnica* – if people do not know about homeopathy already they will view you with suspicion!

As a beginner in homeopathy the first question to ask yourself when someone needs help is 'Am I capable of taking this on?' If you read the three sections below and the fourth on page 108, you will be able to categorize your case and then follow the guidelines for that category. In category one and two contact the emergency services, doctor or homeopath first before thinking about homeopathic treatment. Trying homeopathic remedies while waiting for the doctor to arrive can do no harm. In category three there is less urgency and you can experiment more with homeopathy.

HOW TO USE HOMEOPATHIC REMEDIES

1: Emergency Acute Illnesses

The illness is life-threatening and help is needed urgently. Examples are some injuries, infections, asthma attacks and bleeding, etc.

Professional Help: Make sure the ambulance is on its way and you have done whatever is necessary. You can then give homeopathic treatment yourself while you are waiting, if appropriate, or contact a homeopath
Dose: One tablet of low potency every ten seconds for three doses. One dose of one tablet of potency 30 or higher.
Assessment: These cases require fast action and the right remedy will act within seconds in the most urgent cases. If there is no effect go on to a different remedy.
Also, the effect of one tablet may soon be exhausted so frequent repetitions may be required. You may need to give one tablet of a low potency as often as every few seconds. Even potencies of 30 and over may need repetition every few minutes to maintain the effect.

2: Severe Acute Illnesses

Although not immediately life-threatening the illness is nevertheless serious. Examples are some cases of pneumonia, infections, injuries, etc.

Professional Help: The doctor should be called and also the homeopath, if appropriate. If homeopathy is used then it must be effective quickly. Otherwise antibiotics or other conventional treatment will be necessary.

Dose: One tablet of low potency every three minutes for three doses. One dose of potency 30 or higher.

Assessment: Wait for 30 minutes to two hours depending on the urgency. If there is no improvement use conventional medicine unless it is safe to try another homeopathic remedy. If the treatment is helping, wait. If the condition then gets worse again, or stops getting better, more tablets should be given.

3: Mild Acute Illness

These are illnesses like colds, flu, mild infections and injuries and a whole host of common ailments.

Professional Help: This is not essential as long as the condition does not deteriorate. In this category it is safe for you to give homeopathic treatment while monitoring the patient. Some of these illnesses will be too mild to need treatment, and should be left to take their natural course.

Dose: One tablet of low potency every two hours for four doses. A single dose of potency 30 or higher.

Assessment: Wait for 3 to 24 hours depending on the severity and pace of the illness. Such illnesses as flu where the onset has been gradual may not respond to homeopathy until the following day. On the other hand a child with earache in this category should start to get better after a few hours. If there is no change after these waiting times give a new remedy. If the patient is starting to improve then wait. Repeat the treatment if the improvement wears off or comes to a halt.

For the use of Homeopathic Remedies in Chronic Illnesses refer to chapter 10

TAKING THE ACUTE CASE

Case-taking of acute illnesses concentrates on the here and now of the problem. Whether it is a bruise or pneumonia, the present symptoms will guide you to the right remedy. As far as the choice of remedy is concerned, the patient's normal state of health can be ignored.

When you begin, your patient will usually tell you straight away some basic information. Use that as a starting point to map out the entire geography of the case.

The Aim of Case-Taking

Your aim is to record a complete symptom picture of the patient. A well-taken case is a patient half cured. A well-taken case conveys the individual nature of this particular illness and patient. From the record you will be able to decide the urgency of the case, what kind of illness is involved, and which remedy is required.

The Method of Case-Taking

Begin by observing and absorbing; soak up information like a sponge. Use all your senses, especially your eyes. Write everything down and take your time. Do not at this point ask any of the questions which may occur to you. Have minimum impact on what you are observing. If you step into a pool, the ripples spoil the reflection. Instead, make a note of lines for further enquiry. Concentrate on noticing as much as possible about the patient and his environment. First impressions can be important and can easily be forgotten. The process is patient-centred – put yourself in his position and try to share in his experience.

Record the patient's own words as these give a sense of his inner state. When he has finished speaking, ask him to tell you more about each of the things he has said. Write everything down: its significance may only become clear later. Then ask if there is anything else he has not mentioned. Give him time to think – and then give yourself time to think about what else you need to know. *The Case-Taking Checklist* below gives you an idea of what needs to be covered.

Do not ask these questions directly. Be skilful in obliquely raising a subject that you want to know more about. That way the patient will volunteer information that is important to him and therefore important in the choice of remedy.

Anything that influences a symptom for better or worse is called a *modality*. Modalities are important in the choice of remedy so should always be included in your notes. They tell us the mode of action of the vital energy of the patient. Modalities which apply to the whole patient are called *general modalities* and are especially important.

If there is a pain find out what it feels like and where exactly it is. Find out what makes each symptom better or worse. Also, how did the illness start and did something bring it on? Always ask open questions like 'Is there anything which makes your throat better or worse?' rather than closed questions like 'Do hot drinks help?' Closed questions do not give reliable answers; in particular, the answers do not tell you the intensity of that symptom. In your notes underline the things which are most intense or are stated forcefully by the patient. The most intense things can be underlined three times.

If possible, ask the people close to the patient for their observations. This can help to complete the picture and get the patient's account into perspective.

THE CASE-TAKING CHECKLIST

First, observe and listen to your patient, then pursue lines of investigation arising from that. Finally, look through this list. Do not go through it mechanically; use it to open up new areas of investigation.

The presenting problems All the symptoms the patient has: where each symptom is, how it feels and its modalities.

Is there anything else? Repeat the sequence of enquiry for any other symptoms.

How did the illness begin? Was the illness triggered by something such as getting cold, or by stress? How long did it take to start?

What is the general state of the patient? Is he thirsty? Is he hot or cold? Is he perspiring? Is he hypersensitive to anything? How is the patient affected by the time of day or night, the position he adopts, rest, movement, activities, cold or hot applications, bathing etc? How does his environment affect him, for example temperature, fresh air, draughts, noise, light, smells, food and drinks, the presence of other people, etc? How is his body functioning in terms of restlessness, perspiration, thirst and hunger? Is he wanting or disliking certain foods or drinks? How is he sleeping? What affects his sleep?

Psychological state Get a sense of the patient's mood (eg irritable, angry, sad, changeable, etc.) How is he behaving – is he weepy, aggressive, needy or withdrawn? Is he bad-tempered? Is he worrying? Does he like attention? Does he have fears, anxieties, etc. Is he jumpy, nervous, apathetic, confused or behaving strangely?

When you have recorded everything you can go on to the next stage.

ORGANIZING YOUR NOTES

Homeopathy has a way of introducing order into this apparent chaos of notes. What you have recorded are all *symptoms* of one sort or another. Some are more important than others in the choice of remedy. There are three criteria to apply.

The Hierarchy of Symptoms is the order of importance of human functions in selection of the remedy.

Psychological symptoms concern the patient's emotional and mental state and his behaviour.

General symptoms concern the whole person and the patient will say 'I am . . .' or 'I feel . . .' or 'My whole body is . . .' Two examples are a desire for cold drinks or sweating at night.

Local symptoms are symptoms of one part of the body, for instance a stomachache, a chest infection or a pain. Most of the things the patient tells you at first are in this category.

Strange Symptoms

Symptoms can be common or unusual. In a chest infection it is not surprising if the patient has a cough. A cough that is not bringing up any phlegm is a little more unusual. If the cough is relieved when the patient lies down that is surprising and therefore important.

Intense Symptoms

Symptoms that are intense or stated emphatically you have underlined up to three times.

Now you should make a list of up to about six main symptoms. At the top will be strange psychological symptoms with three underlinings, if there are any. An example would be the patient being convinced he is about to die because he has an earache. The list will continue down the hierarchy with the intense and strange symptoms given priority. If you were to continue right down the list, at the very bottom would be common local symptoms not underlined, such as slight diarrhoea during a tummy upset.

WORKING OUT THE REMEDY

You now have a manageable symptom picture which you can compare with remedy pictures until you find the most similar one. With your necessarily limited knowledge this presents a problem. It would take ages to look through even the small selection of remedies in this book. A short cut is needed. The ideal solution is provided by homeopathic *repertories* which are indexes of all possible symptoms. After each entry there is a list of all the remedies which can cause that symptom in the provings. This does not mean you can give any of those remedies. By cross-referencing, a remedy is found which covers the whole case.

Repertories tend to be huge books. The most popular basic repertory has 1,200 pages and was put together by Dr James Tyler Kent who worked at the turn of the century. Its publication was a landmark in the evolution of homeopathy. The more recent computerization of repertories was another.

These very desirable tools are not often available to beginners. Instead, refer to the list of common illnesses in chapter 7. This is a short cut that works reasonably well. Each illness is followed by a list of possible remedies. Now you have only to look through a handful of remedy pictures.

Each remedy pictures is presented in the hierarchical order to make comparison easier. When comparing the symptom picture of the patient with the remedy picture, be flexible and creative. It is unusual to get a case where all the symptoms fit one remedy. Arriving at the correct remedy is like identifying in a botanical book a flower that is new to you. There always seem to be several possibilities and the decision is complex. First select the remedies that look possible and hopefully there are only about three or four. Rearrange the pieces of the puzzle in your mind until you come up with a combination that matches one remedy clearly.

Your choice of remedy should not be based on one main symptom. A correspondence between case notes and remedy of three really good symptoms is better. Think holistically – consider all the main symptoms. Clarify in your mind the overall themes of the illness such as weakness in one case or intense heat in another. The case as a whole is a picture with certain essential features. Most of the essential features and the overall character of the symptom picture should match the remedy picture. When you have narrowed the possibilities down to a few remedies some of the symptoms lower down the list may help with the final choice. Talking to the patient again may also be helpful. Don't forget to ask about the *modalities* of each symptom and of the whole person. Even if the remedy you choose is not the best one it may help a little, and given as recommended it will do no harm.

GO BY THE SYMPTOMS, NOT THE DISEASE

A homeopathic remedy works by enhancing the vital energy of the patient. The energy of the remedy must correspond to the energy of the patient. To prescribe a remedy you must know the state of that vital energy. This is not visible – it can be understood only by studying the symptoms. This definitely does not mean that homeopathy just treats the symptoms. This criticism sometimes levelled at homeopathy is based on a misunderstanding. The remedy is chosen according to the symptoms but works on a deeper level.

The essence of homeopathic skill lies in assessing the symptoms in order to understand the message from the vital energy. The name of the remedy required is written in the langauge of nature, in the symptoms. The remedy needed does not depend on the name of the disease. Remember that you are treating the patient and the patient will then heal the disease.

Case Example
A friend asks you to help her 12-year-old daughter who has yet another throat infection. You agree to go and see her with your homeopathic remedies and books. First you talk to the mother: you discover that the girl came home from school two days ago feeling hot and headachey, with a sore throat. She developed a

fever and was really ill the following morning. She has been sitting or lying on the settee, eating nothing and drinking a little. Then you go to the patient: she is hot with fever and a little sweaty and flushed. Looking into her mouth you can see that her tonsils are swollen and red – the left being easily visible. She says that her throat hurts a lot. She will drink only cold drinks. When you ask why she replies that she cannot stand hot drinks because they make her throat worse.

You notice that the patient is sitting away from the heater and looks miserable.

You consult the *case-taking checklist* to find out what else you may need to know. Having already covered everything except the patient's general state you ask open questions about that. Your friend, in reply to your question about whether her daughter is better or worse at any time of day or night, says that today and yesterday she was noticeably in more pain first thing in the morning. All other lines of enquiry yield nothing, so your case notes are now complete.

Professional Help: These throat infections can linger for over a week. Your friend already has antibiotics after visiting the doctor yesterday but is reluctant to give them to her daughter. You decide that this is a mild acute illness and it is safe to try homeopathy.

Main Homeopathic Symptoms: < on waking, < left side. Throat pain < hot drinks. The other symptoms are not marked or unusual enough to take into account.

Case Analysis: You consult the list of remedies for throat problems. After writing down the list you look up the remedy pictures. You are looking for a remedy that has the two modalities: < on waking and < left side. Eventually you discover that *lachesis* covers these two symptoms and covers the general character of the case.

Prescription: You have *lachesis* in the 30th potency so you give one tablet and go home, asking your friend to telephone after about six hours. This is a suitable waiting time for a slow-paced acute condition.

Assessment: At that time the patient is reading and is more lively. She says her throat still hurts and she still has a fever. You interpret this as a good reaction so far and decide to await further progress. The next day she is fine. The *lachesis* has worked well as an acute remedy and you suggest to your friend that she should take her daughter to a homeopath for constitutional treatment to prevent any more infections.

Comments: Note that many of the characteristic symptoms of *lachesis* are absent, and this does not matter. The important thing is that what is there fits *lachesis*. There are no psychological symptoms of any significance so general symptoms come to the top of the list. There are two of these, both strongly suggestive of *lachesis*.

The symptoms of importance in choosing the remedy are not the obvious ones, ie, sore throat and fever. A sore throat or fever can be cured by many remedies. The individual symptoms of the patient tell us which is the correct one.

THE GUIDING PRINCIPLES ON POTENCY, DOSE AND REPETITION

In homeopathic evening classes, and at the beginning of college courses, the teachers are often besieged by questions about these basic practicalities. There are so many different recommendations on potency, number of doses and so on that students are confused before they start. This section gives guidance on this. The basic principles are simple and will soon become clear.

One of the most confusing things you can do is take lots of different homeopathic remedies either at the same time or too soon after one another. The results achieved are at best mediocre. If you are treating yourself, discussing things with a friend who is also interested in homeopathy helps to get things into perspective. Treating friends or members of your family is easier, but demands emotional detachment in order to make the right decisions.

The best procedure is outlined in the tables on pages 62, 63 and 108. To go on to a new remedy too soon will stop the previous one working. The waiting time is different in the four categories. In urgent cases the correct homeopathic remedy will work very quickly. It is important not to wait too long before giving a new remedy. In chronic cases, however, it is easy to make the mistake of not waiting long enough.

Once improvement has begun, stop the treatment. Repeat the dose later if the condition gets worse again. Remedies repeated in this way at the right time have a cumulative effect. Remember that homeopathy involves small doses. Successful prescribing includes long periods of time where no treatment at all is given. Vital energy likes to be given a boost then left to work out its own solutions. Give the patient a push in the right direction then wait to see how far he gets. When he is flagging give him another. Sooner or later he will keep going on his own.

When one potency of a remedy has been helping and then no longer works, change to a higher potency of the same remedy.

SELECTING THE POTENCY AND DOSE

Stick to the potencies 6, 6x, 12, 12x (or any potency below 30) at first. When you have read this book and had some experience you may want to use potency 30, which requires fewer repetitions. Do not use higher potencies (200, 1m, 10m, etc) or the LM scale without further training. The higher potencies can occasionally over-stimulate the vital energy and cause unnecessary aggravations. In skin complaints stick to the potencies below 30 for the same reason.

The dose is explained in the four tables above.

ASSESSING THE EFFECTS OF THE TREATMENT

After waiting the required time, record the changes in the condition of the patient. Give particular attention to any changes you notice or are told of in the general state of the patient. At this stage the patient may only just be starting to improve. This may appear as a person being more his usual self, having more energy or being less affected by the illness. Increased discharges, such as coughing up mucus in chest conditions or the appearance of skin eruptions, are also early signs of improvement. Other signs are: in acute illness if the patient goes to sleep, or in chronic illness if old symptoms come back. If one or more of these changes is taking place and the patient is not getting worse in other ways then the remedy is probably working and you should give no more treatment at this point.

You may be in a dilemma here. Is the remedy starting to work, which means it is important not to interfere? Or is the patient not really any better, and in need of a new remedy? It will become clear one way or the other if you follow the guidance in the tables.

In acute illnesses the patient just gets better when given the right remedy – there are no 'aggravations'. These happen only in chronic illnesses where there is a backlog of symptoms and the patient cannot get better without throwing them out. They are severe in only a very small percentage of cases, and sometimes people who know a little about homeopathy anticipate them unnecessarily.

7

Index of Illnesses

THE SECTION CALLED *Working Out the Remedy* in chapter 6 tells you how to use this list. To recap quickly: decide what condition or illness you are treating and find it in this list. Write down the possible remedies and study each one in the remedy pictures which follow. The remedy that matches the symptom picture of the patient is the one to give.

The remedies listed will cover most cases you treat. Sometimes an illness will appear with an unusual symptom picture which is beyond the scope of this small book. I encourage you to get more books if possible.

Some remedies are in capital letters and some in italics, indicating how often they are needed. Those in capital letters are needed most often, those in italics less often and those in ordinary type sometimes. If you are unable to choose between two remedies, give the one that is statistically the most likely. Chronic illnesses have not been included as it is essential that professional help be sought in these cases.

Occasionally a remedy is listed even though it is not described in this book. I have done this if the remedy is an important one for that complaint: you can find out about it from a book in the book list.

Abdominal Problems: see **Digestive Problems**.
Abscesses and Boils (See also **Mastitis**): *arn.*, ars., *bell.*, *hep.* *sulph.*, lach., merc., SIL., sulph.
Allergic Reactions (See also **Hay fever**): ALL. CEP., APIS, ARS.,

euphr., *nat. mur.*, *nux vom.*, *puls.*

Anaemia: see **Weakness.**

Appendicitis: bell., BRY., lach., lyc., merc., *phos.*

Back Problems and Sciatica: *arn.*, *bry.*, *hyper.*, mag. phos., *nux vom.*, *rhus tox.*, ruta, staph.

Bereavement: see **Grief.**

Black Eye: see **Eye Injuries.**

Boils: see **Abscesses and Boils.**

Birth, for recovery from: ARN., bellis, hyper., staph.

Bites and Stings: arn., *bell.*, *apis*, *hyper.*, lach., LEDUM, staph., urt. u.

Bleeding: arn., bell., cal., carbo veg., ferr., ferr. phos., *ham.*, *ipec.*, PHOS.

Blisters: see **Skin problems** or **Burns.**

Blood Poisoning: arn., *ars.*, bapt., echin., *lach.*, pyrog.

Breast Feeding Problems: (See also **Mastitis**) **Cracked or Sore Nipples**: arn., cal., graph., phyt. **Excess Milk**: bell., bry., puls., urt. u. **Insufficient milk**: bell., BRY., puls., *urt u.*

Breathing Difficulties and Asthma Attacks: acon., ant. tart., apis, ARS., bry., *carbo veg.*, cham., cina., *ipecac.*, kali carb., lyc., nux vom., *phos.*, *puls.*, samb., spong.

Broken Bones: ARN., bry., rhus tox., symph.

Bronchitis: see **Chest Problems.**

Bruises: ARN., *bellis.*, hyp., led., ruta., symph.

Burns and Scalds: ars., cal., CANTH., *caust.*, ham., hep. sulph., hyp., *kali bich.*, phos., *urt. u.*

Catarrh: see **Chest Problems, Hay fever.**

Chicken pox: ANT. TART., apis, *ars.*, *bell.*, merc., *puls.*, RHUS TOX.

Chilblains: cham., *bell.*, petr., puls.

Colds: normally straightforward common colds should not be treated. If they persist constitutional treatment is needed.

Colic: *bell.*, bry., *cham.*, *coloc.*, lyc., *mag. phos.*, *nux vom.*, podo., puls., rheum., staph.

Cold Sores: cal., dulc., graph., nat. mur., *rhus tox.*, sep.

Collapse: acon., arn., ars., carbo veg., vera alb.

Conjunctivitis: see **Eye Infections and Inflammations.**

Coughs: see **Chest Problems and Coughs.**

Chest Problems and Coughs: (see also **Allergic Reactions, Breathing Difficulties and Asthma Attacks, Hayfever**): acon., ant. tart., apis., ars., *bell.*, bry., *carbo veg.*, *caust.*, cham., cina, dros., ferr. phos., hep. sulph., ign., *ipec.*, kali carb., lach., *lyc.*, merc., nux vom., PHOS., puls, rhus tox., rumex, sil., spong., sulph

Barking cough: acon., *bell.*, *dros.*, hep. sulph., spong.

Choking cough: hep sulph., IPECAC., kali carb., lach.

Cough < deep breathing: acon., bell., *bry.*, hep. sulph., *kali carb.*, lyc., merc., puls., rhus tox., rumex.

Cough during fever: *acon.*, ars., *bell.*, *bry.*, IPECAC., *kali carb.*, nat. mur., nux vom., phos., sabad.

Cough > raising phlegm: hep., ipec., lach., phos.

Cough < talking: bell., caust., *dros.*, hep. sulph., lach., merc., PHOS., rumex., spong.

Cough with rattling in chest: ant. tart., bell., bry., *caust.*, *ipecac.*, nux vom., puls., sil.

Croupy cough: ACON., ars., *bell.*, cina., *hep. sulph.*, lach., *phos.*, rumex., samb., spong.

Painful breathing: acon., *bell.*, BRY., carbo veg., *caust.*, dros., phos., nux vom.

Painful cough: all. cep., BRY., caust., merc., *nux vom.*, *phos.*, rhus tox.

Cramp: bell., cina., *coloc.*, *mag. phos.*, *nux vom.*

Cricked Neck: see **Stiff Neck.**

Croup: see **Coughs, croupy.**

Cuts: see **Wounds.**

Cystitis, Urethritis: ars., apis, bell., CANTH., caust., equis., *merc.*, nat. mur., *nux vom.*, puls., SARS., *staph.*, *sulph.*

Dehydration: Carbo veg., CHIN., phos., puls., *staph.*

Dentistry, after: ARN., hyp., led., nux vom., ruta., phos., staph.

Dermatitis: see **Skin Problems.**

Diaper Rash: see **Nappy Rash.**

Diarrhoea: see **Digestive Problems.**

Digestive Problems: ant. tart., ARS., bell., *bry.*, carbo veg., *cham.*, coloc., gels., *ipecac.*, kali carb., LYC., mag. phos., merc., nat. mur., NUX VOM., op., podo., phos., puls., sulph., vera. a.

Colic: bell., cham., coloc., mag. phos., nux vom., staph.

From food poisoning: ars., carbo veg., lach., lyc., merc., puls.

From overindulgence: ant. c., ars., ipecac., lyc., *nux vom.*, sulph.

From emotional upsets or nerves: arg. nit., cham., coloc., gels., ign., lyc., puls., op., staph.

From teething: ars., bell., CHAM., cina., *rheum.*

Traveller's tummy: *ars.*, lyc., nux vom., puls.

With wind: arg. nit., carbo veg., *lyc.*, nux vom.

With chill: ars., phos., verat. a.

Dislocations: arn., bry., rhus tox., ruta.

Drowning: ant. tart.

Ear Infections and Earaches: *acon.*, *bell.*, cham., *ferr. phos.*, hep. sulph., lach., lyc., *merc.*, phos., *puls.*, *sil.*

Emotional Problems: (see also **Grief** and **Nervousness**) The following remedies may also be needed in any patient where these emotions figure prominently.

> **Anger**: CHAM., *coloc.*, *hep.*, ign., NUX VOM., *staph.*, *stram.*
>
> **Anxiety**: acon., *Arg. nit.*, ARS., bry., caust., *gels.*, lyc., puls.
>
> **Being critical or fussy**: ARS, *nux vom.*, verat. a.
>
> **Dislike of sympathy**: ign., *nat. mur.*, sep.
>
> **Excitement**: *coff.*, gels., ign., phos., puls., staph.
>
> **Fright or Fear**: ACON., *ars.*, bell., ign., op., *phos.*, puls., *stram.*
>
> **Jealousy**: *apis*, ign., LACH., nux vom., puls., staph.
>
> **Sadness**: gels., ign., nat. mur., puls.
>
> **Weeping**: apis, ign., PULS.

Eye Infections and Inflammations: *acon.*, *all. cep.*, *apis*, *ars.*, *bell.*, bry., *euphr.*, lyc., *merc.*, nux vom., *puls.*, *staph.*

Eye Injuries: *arn.*, *cal.*, euphr., *led.*, staph., SYMPH.

Exhaustion: ant. tart., bry., carbo veg., gels., merc., nux vom., phos.

Fainting or Faintness: carbo veg., op., puls.

Fever: ACON, apis, *ars.*, BELL, *bry.*, cham., FERR. PHOS., *gels.*, *lyc.*, *merc.*, *nat. mur.*, *nux vom.*, *phos.*, *puls.*, rhus tox.

Flu: acon., ars., bell., *bry.*, *eup. perf.*, ferr. phos., GELS., *nux vom.*, phos., puls., rhus tox.

Food Poisoning: see **Digestive Problems.**

Foreign bodies: hep. sulph., *sil.*

Fractures: see **Broken Bones.**

Gastro-enteritis: see **Digestive Problems.**

German measles: acon., BELL., *ferr. phos.*, *puls.*

Gout: *bell.*, *led.*, puls., *urt. u.*

Grazes: see **Wounds.**

Grief: IGN., nat mur., *puls.*, *staph.*

Gum Boils: see **Abscesses and Boils.**

Hay fever: ALL. CEP., *ars.*, euphr., nat. mur., nux vom., puls., sabad., sil.

Headaches and Migraines: ars., bell., *bry.*, gels., ign., lach., lyc., nat. mur., *nux vom.*, phos., puls.

Head Injuries: ARN., hyp., led.

Heartburn: see **Digestive Problems.**

Heat Exhaustion, Sunstroke: acon., BELL., bry., gels., *glon.*, lach., nat. mur., puls., verat. a.

Heat Rash: see **Skin Problems.**

Hepatitis: ars., bell., bry., *chel.*, LYC., merc., nux vom., phos.

Herpes Simplex: see **Cold Sores.**

Herpes Zoster: see **Shingles.**

Hives: see **Skin Problems.**

Housemaid's Knee: see **Injuries.**

Immunization, ill effects of: acon., apis., ars., *bell.*, merc.

Impetigo: ars., graph., merc., rhus tox., sulph.

Infections: see under part of body infected

Influenza: see **Flu**

Injuries: (See also **Bites and Stings, Broken Bones, Burns and Scalds, Eye Injuries, Head Injuries, Wounds**) ARN., bellis., bry., *cal.*, hyper., *led.*, phos., staph., *symph.*, *rhus tox.*, ruta. Of joints: *bry.*, *rhus tox.*

Hiccoughs: ign., mag. phos, nux vom.

Homesickness: *bry.*, ign., merc., staph.

Insomnia: see **Sleeplessness.**

Jet lag: *arn.*, *cocc.*, gels.

Joint Injuries: see **Injuries.**

Kidney Problems: APIS, *ars.*, BELL., *berb.*, bry., *canth.*, lyc., puls.

Laryngitis: acon., bell., dros., gels., phos., spong.

Malaria: chin., *nat. mur.*, nux vom.

Mastitis (and **Breast Abscesses**): apis, BELL., BRY., hep., lach., lyc., merc., phos., puls., *phyt.*, sil.

Measles: acon., *apis*, ars., BELL., bry., euphr., *ferr. phos.*, gels., *puls.*

Meningitis: acon., *apis*, BELL., bry., lach., merc., phos., stram.

Migraines: see **Headaches and Migraines.**

Morning Sickness: see **Nausea in Pregnancy.**

Motion Sickness: see **Travel Sickness.**

Mumps: acon., apis, ars., *bell.*, bry., cham., lach., lyc., *merc.*, phyt., pilo., *puls.*, rhus tox.

Nails, Inflamed or Infected: bell., hep., sil.

Nappy Rash: apis, ars., *bell.*, cal.

Nausea and Vomiting: see **Digestive Problems.**

In Pregnancy: ipecac., kreos., *nux vom.*, *puls.*, *sep.*, tab.

Nervousness (anticipation): *Arg. nit.*, *gels.*, *lyc.*

Nosebleeds: acon., arn., bell., bry., *ferr. phos.*, ham., lach., led., *phos.*

Operations: see **Surgery, after.**

Overexertion: arn., rhus tox.

Period Pains: bell., caul., cham., cimic., coloc., lach., mag. phos.

Pleurisy: see **Chest Problems.**

Pneumonia: see **Chest Problems.**

Prickly heat: see **Skin Problems.**

Rashes: see **Skin Problems.**

Retention of urine: acon., *apis.*, arn., ars., bell., *caust.*, op.

Ringworm: graph., sep., sulph.

Rubella: see **German Measles.**

Scalds: see **Burns and Scalds.**

Scarlet Fever and Scarlatina: apis, BELL., bry., cham., lach., lyc., merc., phos., rhus tox.

Sciatica: see **Back Problems.**

Scratches: see **Wounds.**

Septicaemia: see **Blood Poisoning,**

Shingles: apis., ARS., hep., lach., merc., RHUS TOX.

Shock: acon., ARN., ign., op.

Sinusitis see **Colds.**

Skin Problems: ars., apis, bell., cham., graph., hep., merc., rhus tox., urt. u.

Sleeplessness: acon., ars., cham., *coff.*, *ign.*, nux vom., phos.

Splinters: see **Foreign Bodies.**

Sports Injuries: see **Injuries.**

Sprains, Strains see **Injuries.**

Stings: see **Bites and Stings.**

Stomach upsets: see **Digestive Problems.**

Stress: see **Emotional Problems.**

Styes: apis, graph., lyc., merc., puls., *staph.*

Suffocation: Ant. tart., carbo veg., op.

Sunburn: bell., cal.

Sunstroke: see **Heat Exhaustion.**

Surgery, after: ARN., *bellis.*, cal., *staph.*, *stront. carb.*

Teething: acon., bell., CHAM., cina., ign., kreos., puls., rheum.

Tennis Elbow: see **Injuries.**

Tetanus: arn., HYP., *led.*

Throat Problems: acon., *apis.*, ars., BELL., bry., ferr. phos., hep.

sulph., ign., LACH., *lyc.*, MERC., nux vom., puls., rhus tox., sil.

Thrush, Oral: ant. tart., *bor.*, cham., merc.

   Genital: *bor.*, merc., nat. mur., sep.

Tiredness: see **Exhaustion.**

Tonsillitis: see **Throat Problems.**

Toothache: acon., arn., bell., cham., coff., kreos., MERC., *nux vom.*, puls., STAPH.

Travel Sickness: arn., cocc., nux vom., petr., sep., tabac.

Ulcers, Skin: see **Skin Problems.**

   Mouth: ars., lyc., MERC.

Urethritis: see **Cystitis.**

Urticaria: see **Skin Problems.**

Vaccination: see **Immunization.**

Vomiting: see **Digestive Problems.**

Weakness: see **Exhaustion.**

Whooping Cough: ars., bell., DROS., ferr. phos., lyc., puls., rumex., spong.

Wounds: apis, cal., *hyp.*, *led.*, staph.

X-Ray and Radiation Effects: rad. brom., ruta.

8

First Aid Remedies

The conditions covered in this section are all kinds of physical injury, including shock. For example: bruising, sprains and strains, broken bones, bleeding, cuts, puncture wounds, grazes and burns. The remedies are those included in the first-aid kit in chapter 5.

Arnica (the Fall Herb, a mountain flower)
Arnica is the essential first aid remedy. It is required for many cases of physical injury to any part of the body, from mild bruising to serious trauma and associated shock. The patient may have been kicked in a football match or have only just survived a serious car accident. Arnica may also be needed after dentistry, surgical operations and childbirth if bruising, soreness and possibly shock predominate.

Using arnica is an easy introduction to homeopathic prescribing. It is almost a routine prescription for this kind of physical injury – unless the symptoms point to another remedy in this section. For most other injuries and for illness in general it is necessary to work out the right remedy for each case individually. Here are some indications for arnica:

- Injuries where bruising predominates. For minor bruises that need treatment use arnica cream.
- The affected area is usually sore and made worse by touch.
- In shock, patients may insist that they are perfectly all right when they are obviously not.
- The typical state of shock: confusion, unclear speech, even unconsciousness.

Conditions that can be healed by arnica if it is indicated by the symptoms include: bruising, sprains (damage to a joint), strains (damaged muscle), dislocations, broken bones, bleeding (including internal bleeding), nosebleeds, concussion, stroke (cerebrovascular accident), injuries to eyes, teeth and gums, testicular injuries and lingering effects of old injuries.

Once, on holiday on the island of Crete, as I pulled my luggage out of the storage compartment of a bus, a very heavy metal spare part fell on my ankle. By the time I had limped to a hotel I was in agony and I automatically took arnica. I fell asleep in no time and was more or less better by the following morning. Such miraculous assistance engenders a profound sense of gratitude to the little flower itself and to homeopathy in general.

Do not apply arnica cream or lotion to broken skin as it may cause inflammation.

If arnica is not working well enough in an injury, consider ruta, rhus tox., bellis, bryonia, ledum and symphytum.

Ruta (Rue, a garden herb)
If the injury is sustained where bone is close to the skin, ruta is usually required. It is the remedy for damage to the surfaces of bones.

Ruta may also be required for sprains and strains, like arnica. The injured part may hurt more if lain on, and can feel lame, weak or broken. The pain tends to make the patient restless.

Ruta is often needed for injuries to knees, ankles and wrists, for tennis elbow and for eyestrain (and associated headache). Michelangelo drank rue tea after a hard day's painting.

Bellis (Daisy)
The name is short for 'day's eye'. The pupil of the daisy's eye is golden yellow like the sun it welcomes each day.

Some cases needing this remedy will be similar to those needing arnica – bruising, falls, etc. So if arnica is not working, consider bellis. In addition, bellis has several quite specific uses of its own. It is the first choice for the following:

- Where deeper tissues are affected, such as the abdomen or pelvis, especially after surgical operations.
- Problems which have arisen from getting chilled or wet when hot, (like rhus tox.) or eating or drinking something cold.

- Lumps remaining long after an injury.
- Injuries to the breasts.

You may have noticed after cutting the lawn how quickly the bright little daisies are flowering again. In medicine, as in nature, bellis has the power of rapid recovery if the symptoms fit the bellis picture. The interesting features of the sources of homeopathic remedies often give hints of their uses.

Rhus tox. (Poison Ivy, a North American climbing shrub)
Rhus tox. is a 'polychrest' – a remedy with many uses. As well as for injuries, it may be needed in throat infections, childhood illnesses, arthritis and many other conditions (see chapter 8).

Sprains and strains are the types of injury where rhus tox. is most often indicated by the symptoms. The pain or stiffness is nearly always relieved by movement – but getting going is difficult; hence the title 'the rusty gate remedy'. In homeopathic terminology, *beginning to move aggravates, continued motion ameliorates*. A sprained ankle will perhaps hurt most the following morning, or whenever the patient begins to move after being at rest – so he or she may like to keep the joint moving all the time to prevent it seizing up. Sometimes the patient will be so weak or exhausted he or she cannot move, even though movement would help. Another lead towards rhus tox. is an aggravation from getting wet or from damp conditions. Hot bathing and warmth in any form, help.

Arnica and rhus tox. are the two remedies most often called for after overexertion, such as straining to lift something too heavy, or too long in the garden or the gym. (Arnica cases are not relieved by continued motion.)

Bryonia (White Bryony, a wild European climbing plant)
Bryonia is the opposite of the rhus tox.; everything is nearly always *made worse by movement*, in some cases even the slightest movement. The patient usually wants to keep perfectly still. Pressure also helps to relieve the pain so the patient may be holding the affected part or lying on it or may like tight bandaging.

The first-aid cases covered by bryonia are usually broken bones and sprains. Broken ribs often call for this remedy. Like rhus tox., bryonia is a polychrest so there is more about it in the next chapter.

Symphytum (Comfrey, or Knitbone)

This is another remedy which has proved invaluable in some specific circumstances. We know from centuries of use unpotentized as a herb that comfrey can help in many injuries – especially in injuries to bone or cartilage when other remedies are not doing the trick.

- It may be needed in comminuted fractures (when there is bone broken into little pieces) or injuries to hands or feet where small bones, cartilage, tendons and ligaments may all be damaged together.
- For injuries to the eyeball where there is no bleeding.
- For cracked bones, or pain in broken bones that are slow to heal. It will speed up the healing.

Hypericum (St John's Wort)

This herb grows in the wild and in gardens. The leaves are full of tiny holes, visible as bright dots when you hold the leaves up to the light. When you crush the flowers your fingers are left stained red, as if with blood. Here is the *doctrine of signatures* telling us that hypericum is good for puncture wounds and bleeding.

Think of hypericum for injuries to parts rich in nerves, such as fingers (tips especially), toes, nail beds, the spine (especially the coccyx, the 'tail bone'), spinal chord and brain, mouth and lips. Examples of these are fingers hit by a hammer or trapped in a door. Also for injuries anywhere which are inordinately painful (showing that nerves are involved) such as nerve pains after dentistry.

Think of either hypericum (or ledum, see below) for puncture wounds where the flesh has been pierced by a nail, splinter or a sting or a bite (of plant, insect or animal) or after surgery or injections (especially an epidural). The wound may be inflamed or infected, and pain shooting from the wound up the nerves is a strong pointer to the need for hypericum. Successful homeopathic treatment of these wounds automatically helps prevent tetanus or other infections. In tetanus, where the wound has affected the nervous system, hypericum may help.

Ledum (Wild Rosemary)

Use ledum first for puncture wounds, bites and stings (as described under hypericum) unless another remedy is indicated by the symptoms. This remedy may also be needed for a black eye and occasionally for other dark coloured bruises when arnica can do no more. The wounded area may feel cold, yet sometimes cold applications help with the pain. Apis may also be needed for bites and stings which are relieved by cold applications, but in apis the wound feels hot.

Calendula (Marigold)
This is the main remedy for skin injuries – grazes, cuts or torn skin. It is excellent as a cream for soothing childrens' minor skin problems. Larger wounds should be kept completely clean, so do not apply cream or ointment. Calendula is also available as a lotion (which should be diluted as instructed on the bottle to prevent stinging) and as tablets. Use the tablets when the injury is more severe, to encourage healing from within, as long as no other remedy is indicated by the symptoms. After a tooth extraction usually arnica is needed first. Give calendula, both as tablets and a mouthwash, when bleeding persists.

Staphysagria (Stavesacre or larkspur, a delphinium)
Occasionally needed for minor skin injuries, stings and bites, this remedy is more often needed for serious injuries or after operations. The wound is hypersensitive, as if the nerves are raw. After an operation the whole body may be reacting as if to an invasion. Any operation could produce this reaction, but especially stretching of body openings and abdominal surgery. Information on this remedy will also be found below in the *Acute Remedy Pictures* below.

Treatment for Burns Various creams and lotions are available for minor burns: they are usually based on a mixture of calendula, hypericum and urtica urens (small stinging nettle). Urtica can also be taken as tablets if the pain persists. For more serious burns with blistering or deeper damage, the usual remedy is *cantharis* (Spanish Fly, see *Acute Remedy Pictures*) taken as tablets. This usually works marvellously to reduce pain, promote healing and help prevent scarring. If the patient is in a state of shock, give arnica first, then soon go on to a specific burn medicine. *Causticum* is often required for deep burns which are very painful, and *kali bichromicum* for deeper burns that have penetrated into the tissues, like ulcers. For electrical burns give *phosphorus*. For X-ray burns, sunbed burns, some severe cases of sunburn and for radiation effects generally give *radium bromide*.

9

Remedies for Common Illnesses

THIS CHAPTER GIVES descriptions of the acute conditions where each remedy is required. Each remedy picture describes the illnesses which the remedy can cure and the physical and psychological state of the patient. The remedy will work if its symptom picture is similar to the symptom picture of the patient. To find this similar remedy the whole of the patient must be taken into account. Chapter 6 explains this: it is essential to read that chapter first.

Remember that these remedy pictures are derived from the provings. A large number of people took part in these, and a huge number of symptoms is included. Your patient will have only a few of these and no one symptom is essential. For example, we read in the description of *Aconite: Causation: getting chilled (or, more rarely, overheated), cold wind. Fright, shock, life-threatening ordeals such as mugging, rape, etc.* Aconite could still be the right remedy if the illness was not caused by any of these things.

To continue with the example: if the patient you are treating became ill suddenly with a high fever and is flushed red in the face one minute then pale the next, but is not agitated or tense and has no other aconite characteristics, you should still give aconite. Three clear similarities is good – more is very reassuring – but you may sometimes have to base your prescriptions on less. Each patient will only ever have part of the whole symptom picture of the remedy, but the whole of the essential quality of the patient should be there in the remedy picture.

The information is given in the following order: *psychological state, general characteristics, modalities, causation, other features etc., illnesses.* The similarity between the patient and the remedy in psychological state, general characteristics and modalities is most important. The illness you are treating will usually appear in the list at the end but if not, that does not matter. This is a crucial difference between homeopathy and orthodox medicine. Using homeopathic medicines involves looking at disease in a radically new way.

These descriptions cover use of the remedies for acute ill-ness. For chronic illness refer to the next chapter. The chronic remedy pictures include some of the information given here, together with more information about personality types and constitutional characteristics such as food preferences etc.

Aconite (Monk's Hood, Aconitum Napellus)

Many times I have been called by distressed parents because a child developed earache, croup or a fever or another acute illness suddenly in the night. If the child got cold the previous day aconite is often the remedy.

Psychological State: Fearful – even believing death is imminent. The condition can seem life-threatening to the patient. Sudden frightening illnesses.

General Characteristics: Aconite complaints tend to come on suddenly, and be intense. The patient is usually tense, restless and sensitive. There may be tossing and turning; the pain or the illness seem unbearable, the patient demands urgent relief. For example, a baby could be crying frantically.

Modalities: Worse at night, from dry cold wind, jarring, noise, music, touch and lying on the affected side. Better from perspiration, uncovering and open air.

Other Features: Burning fever, possibly with phases of coldness or paleness. Face alternately red and pale. One cheek red. Dry, barking or croupy cough. The main remedy for croup. Dry eyes, mouth, etc. Intense thirst. Frantic agitation. Violent palpitations. Newborn babies in a state of shock, or with retention of urine.

Causation: Getting chilled (or, more rarely, overheated), cold wind. Fright, shock, life-threatening ordeals such as mugging and rape.

Illnesses: Shock, fevers, coughs, croup, earache, asthma attacks, breathlessness, infections, fevers, childhood illnesses.

Allium Cepa (Red Onion)

Allium cepa is a constituent of many combination remedies used for hay fever. These combinations can work to some extent because of the 'blunderbuss' effect. A remedy chosen more exactly will work better. This one is made from onion and everyone knows what that can cause – and cure.

General Characteristics: Inflammations with lots of watery discharges. Burning or smarting pains.

Modalities: Worse in warm rooms. Better in the open air, in cool rooms.

Other Features: The nasal discharge burns, but the tears do not (the reverse of euphrasia). Coughing and sneezing together. One nostril runny. Colds in damp weather.

Illnesses: Allergies, hay fever, eye inflammations and coughs.

Antimonium Tartaricum (Antimony potassium tartrate)

Ant. tart. is not made from insects and pastry but from black antimony which sinks to the bottom of the container when it is prepared chemically and sticks there. It gets its name from Tartarus, the mythological lowest region of the underworld, from which it is almost impossible to rise. Part of the symptom picture is of mucus flooding the lungs which cannot be coughed up.

General Characteristics: Drowsiness, sinking strength. Respiratory and digestive complaints together. Clammy sweat. (The face may be pale and sunken; the lips may be going blue.)

Modalities: Better in an upright position, after raising mucus. Worse from warmth, milk and when given attention.

Respiratory Problems: The cough is unproductive so the chest is rattling with mucus, causing difficulty in breathing. Vomiting of mucus. Asphyxia of newborn babies. Suffocation, drowning and choking.

Digestive Problems: Nausea which comes and goes. Indigestion from milk in children. Babies with feeding problems and angry crying. Forcible vomiting, or ineffectual efforts to vomit.

Other Features: Complaints of children and the elderly. Some cases of chicken pox, including ones where the rash is not appearing properly.

Illnesses: Respiratory problems, stomach upsets, chicken pox.

Apis (the Honey Bee, Apis Mellifica)

This remedy is made from the honey bee. Bee stings cause swelling and burning pains, which gives hints to the use of the remedy. Further insights come from the behaviour of bees: their busy lives, their aggressive reaction to interference and their jealous guarding of the queen. The hives have a special cooling system to prevent overheating.

Psychological State: Sad, weepy, disappointed. Jealous. A 'queen bee' state of mind; touchy, fussy and demanding. Clumsiness, especially dropping things.

General characteristics: Puffy swellings, sometimes like sacks of water; tight, itchy, painful or red swellings often near the eyes or of the face or throat. Burning or stinging pains. Sudden pains making the patient cry out. Complaints are often worse on, or start on, the right side.

Modalities: Worse after sleep, from touch, from heat in any form. Worse 3–5pm. Better from cold applications, cold drinks, cold air, open air.

Causation: Emotions like jealousy and anger.

Fever: High fever without thirst, with sleepiness, with sensitive skin. One part hot, another part cold.

Respiratory Problems: When caused by overheating, or accompanied by heat or chill or constricted throat. Panting, gasping for breath, needing the windows open.

Other features: Symptoms that resemble the effects of a bee sting. Meningitis; the shrieking in the apis symptom picture caused by the pain, or coming during sleep or unconsciousness, is like the 'brain cry' of meningitis. Hydrocephalus. Scanty urine.

Illnesses: Allergic reactions, inflammations and infections of any part of the body (including joints and kidneys), respiratory conditions, fever, swellings, oedema, serous effusion, hives, measles, cystitis and any illness where the symptoms indicate apis.

Arsenicum Album (White Arsenic, Arsenic trioxide)

There is more on this remedy in the case study on page six.

Psychological State: The arsenicum patient is typically anxious, restless, critical and fastidious. He tends to be a difficult patient – hard to please and intolerant of disorder or mess. He is often worried about his illness and fears the worst, needing company and lots of reassurance. The restlessness makes him toss and turn in bed, or move around the house, even to try different beds. Fast movement can have a calming effect.

General Characteristics: The patient is usually cold, restless and anxious. Burning pains, but the patient still loves heat. Burning discharges (for example causing sore nostrils in colds and sore anus in diarrhoea). Dryness of the mouth with thirst for frequent sips of liquid (although the patient can also be thirsty for larger amounts). Exhaustion. Illnesses producing sudden or extreme weakness.

Modalities: Worse from about midnight to 2am, from cold, from exertion, from sight or smell of food. Better from warm food or drink and from cool air to the head.

Causation: Food poisoning, cold food, getting chilled, insecurity.

Fever: With great sensitivity to cold. With the feeling of heat internally and cold externally, or vice versa. Burning (or icy coldness) in the blood vessels.

Digestion: Diarrhoea that can be offensive smelling, burning and exhausting. Vomiting. The vomiting can be frequent and very easily induced, eg straight after drinking, possibly even the smallest amount (phosphorus also has this symptom), on moving, during perspiration.

Other Features: Blackness; of skin, lips, of vomited material etc. Corpse-like body odour. Pale face, haggard expression. Asthma attacks where the patient cannot bear to stay in bed.

Illnesses: Anxiety states, diarrhoea, stomach upsets, food poisoning, all sorts of infections, inflammations and fevers, common colds, any condition presenting the symptom picture of arsenicum.

Belladonna (Deadly Nightshade)

My first experience of the dramatic speed with which belladonna can sometimes work was one night when my daughter woke up suddenly with a high fever. She was very hot, and obviously having hallucinations. She had gone to bed in a cold room with wet hair.

Psychological State: May be listless, for example during a fever. Also can have hypersensitive senses, or be wild and delirious – behaving violently, muttering or seeing monsters, frightening faces, etc. Frightful nightmares.

General Characteristics: Sudden violent conditions. Heat, bright redness and throbbing of the whole patient or the affected part. Complaints accompanied by shiny or staring eyes, dilated pupils, or flushed face. The patient may radiate heat. A desire for lemonade or lemon juice. Muscular spasms from cramps and twitches to febrile convulsions (convulsions brought on by high fever).

Modalities: Worse at 3pm, on the right side of the body (eg earache), from light, noise and jar; also from allowing the affected part to hang downwards or from lying on the painful side. Better lying on the abdomen or bending backwards.

Fever: With photophobia, with hot head and cold hands and feet. With delirium or hallucinations. With sweat on covered parts.

Other Features: Sensitive head. Congestion of the head. Full hard pulse. Jerking in sleep. May be the remedy for any infections from cystitis to earache (including chest and throat infections).

Illnesses: Fevers, inflammations and infections of all kinds; childhood illnesses, coughs, delirious fevers, headaches, sunstroke, photophobia, abdominal cramps, colic, muscular spasms, inflamed boils, nappy rash, sunburn and all complaints where the symptom picture of belladonna is present.

Bryonia (White Bryony, Wild Hops)

Children can throw up very high fevers (for which, incidentally, belladonna is often the indicated remedy). It is a sign of their high levels of vital energy and their powerful immune response.

The second fever that my daughter had did not call for belladonna. She was very very thirsty, and was delirious, saying 'I want to go home'. This strange psychological symptom of wanting to go home, even though she already was at home, suggested the remedy bryonia. Her great thirst confirmed this.

Psychological State: Bryonia patients tend to want to be left alone rather than be fussed over. They can be irritable, for instance, if asked questions. They want stillness of mind as well as of body and do not want to think or respond. Usually not talkative, they can however be worried about business or financial matters and talk about them. This applies when they are delirious and they can be obsessed with getting back to work or to their studies.

General Characteristics: There are two important themes in bryonia cases: aggravation of the condition from any movement and dryness (of mucous membranes, lips, mouth, etc). Even the slightest motion may be painful, for example moving the eyes during a headache. In back problems the patient will keep every part of his body still. In chest problems coughing, and even breathing, can be painful.

Other remedies can have this sensitivity to motion (though usually not so intensely) so try to confirm the choice of bryonia with other symptoms; thirst for large amounts of liquid, often drunk all in one go; sticking or stitching pains.

Modalities: Worse from motion, warm rooms, warmth generally, in the evening, especially at 9pm, after eating. Better from pressure applied to the painful part, holding the chest when coughing, lying on the painful side, keeping still.

Causation: Financial worries, exposure to cold.

Other Features: Constipation with large dry stool. Constipation on holiday. Digestive problems during fevers or relieved by warm drinks. Gradual onset of illness (unlike belladonna). Fever with changeable sequence of heat, chill and sweat, perhaps occurring in the autumn. Increased perspiration in the open air.

Illnesses: May be the remedy indicated in a wide range of illnesses similar to belladonna. Dry pleurisy. Mastitis. Appendicitis. Influenza. Muscle, back and joint problems.

Cantharis (Spanish Fly)
This remedy is used mainly for urinary infections and burns (see previous chapter).

Psychological State: Restless and frenzied because of the pain.

General Characteristics: Burning pains. Thirst with no desire to actually drink.

Modalities: Cold applications relieve. Coffee aggravates.

Cystitis: Urgent frequent desire to urinate. Burning pains before, during or after urination, but most often near the beginning.

Illnesses: Cystitis, urethritis, kidney problems.

Carbo vegetabilis (Charcoal)

This remedy shows how the substance which the remedy is made from is similar to the patient who needs the remedy. Charcoal is made by burning wood without air. The patient also feels deprived of air, having a hunger for cold fresh air. In charcoal production impurities are driven off in the smoke. The patient also produces noxious fumes, from both ends.

Psychological State: The patient can be unmotivated and not care about his or her state.

General Characteristics: Weak and cold, with cold sweat – yet a strong desire for cold air, and sometimes the patient wants to be fanned. Cold breath, cold tongue. Weak pulse. Pale or blue face and skin. Sluggish weakness, over-relaxation: of the whole person or of lungs or circulation. Feeling full and heavy. Difficulty in breathing. This remedy could be needed in a prolonged illness or a sudden collapse.

Modalities: Better: air (cold and fresh); fanning; passing wind. Worse: exertion; fatty or rich food; in the evening.

Causation: Shock, poisoning (especially by gases), accident, injury, bleeding.

Indigestion: After overindulgence. Fullness and bloating with unpleasant belching or flatulence. Headache with indigestion.

Other Features: Slow bleeding of dark (venous) blood. Puffy purplish swollen tissue.

Illnesses: Indigestion, collapse, bleeding, breathing problems, coughs, slow recovery from illness or surgery.

Causticum

This mineral compound was created by Hahnemann from slaked lime and potash. It is unknown outside homeopathy.

Psychological State: Tired and weak. Crying easily.

General Characteristics: Trembling, weakness or paralysed feeling.

Modalities: Worse from cold or dry air. Better: from cold drinks, cold applications.

Cough: The patient cannot cough up the mucus, or involuntarily swallows it down again. Coughing or sneezing may cause incontinence. Cough relieved by sips of water. Hoarse or weak voice. The chest feels raw and sore.

Face: Neuralgia or paralysis after getting cold, usually on the right side.

Other Features: Frequent swallowing. Burning pains. Burns: severe or chemical, often with blisters. (Slaked lime burns the skin.)
Illnesses: coughs, paralysis (eg of bladder, facial muscles), loss of voice, cramps, burns.

Chamomilla (German Chamomile)

Chamomilla is the well-known saviour of many teething or colicky babies, and their parents – except when it doesn't work, and cina, nux vom., coloc., rheum, or another remedy is needed. Chamomilla is over-used because of its reputation. If it is given every time a baby is distressed, it loses its effectiveness.
Psychological State: Irritable, excitable, whining, impossible to placate. Great sensitivity to pain. Pain causes anger. Demanding something then rejecting it. Everything feels oppressive.
General Characteristics: Unbearable pains. Sweating or fainting from pain. Pain with numbness. Distressed infants or babies who are whinging or crying frantically, often during teething or colic and need to be carried all the time. Sleeplessness from pain.
Modalities: Worse from attention, touch, being out in wind, warmth, night-time, 9am or 9pm. Better from being carried.
Causation: Teething. Anger. Drinking coffee.
Other Features: One red cheek. Sour body odour. Green diarrhoea, perhaps smelling of rotten eggs. Diarrhoea in teething babies. Labour pains sometimes need chamomilla. Toothache after getting angry.
Illnesses: Teething, stomach upsets, colic, diarrhoea, ear problems, fevers, sleeplessness.

Cina (Wormseed)

There is a rather extreme cina case in chapter 3. This remedy will cure fevers, coughs and digestive problems if they are associated with the touchy emotional state of cina. The patient is usually a child who gets angry at any interference, even loving attention.

Coffea (Coffee)

Coffea cures states of over-excitement, mental hyperactivity, and acute senses. It is often used for sleeplessness if the symptoms fit. It also covers toothache if the pain responds well to cold water held near the tooth. See also page 38.

Colocynth (Bitter Cucumber)
The main feature of this remedy is cramping pains which make the patient double up. The pains may be relieved by leaning over something hard or by pressing on the abdomen. If coloc. is the remedy for colic, then anger is usually the trigger of the problem, or at least the patient is very irritable because of the pain.

Drosera (Sundew, a carnivorous plant)
This remedy is used for whooping cough or other violent coughs with retching or gagging. The cough may be accompanied by a tickle in the throat, nosebleeds or blueness of the face, and the hours after midnight are the worst time.

Eupatorium Perfoliatum (Boneset)
The American pioneers used this remedy for 'breakbone fever'. If flu is accompanied by pains in the bones (possibly feeling as if the bones are broken) then eup. perf. may be the remedy. There can be a desire for ice-cold water, and early morning tends to be the worst time.

Euphrasia (Eyebright)
According to *the doctrine of signatures* the medicinal uses of a plant can be observed in its appearance and habits. Eyebright flowers have purple and yellow spots which resemble bloodshot or diseased eyes. It is used when eye symptoms predominate in such conditions as hay fever, measles and allergic reactions. The tears or discharges from the eyes are burning to the skin; the nasal discharge is bland. Mucous membranes of the eyes, nose or mouth can be swollen, red and discharging.

Ferrum Phosphorica (Iron phosphate)
Ferrum phos. is sometimes needed in fevers, infections and

inflammatory illnesses which do not have the intensity of aconite or belladonna. In fact this remedy should be considered in illnesses of that kind which do not seem to fit any other remedy very clearly.

Psychological State: Usually tired and indifferent, but possibly quite alert even when ill; sometimes even cheerful and lively.

General Characteristics: Gradual onset. Blood-streaked discharges, or easy bleeding (eg, from nose, gums) during fevers etc. Throbbing.

Modalities: Better from gentle movement. Worse on right side from touch, jar, exertion, standing, and at 4–6am.

Other Features: Pale, but possibly flushing easily. Clearly defined red cheeks. Pale mucous membranes. Hard dry tickling cough with sore throat. Maybe needed after arnica in injuries involving bleeding or bruising. Earaches belladonna does not cure.

Illnesses: Coughs and colds, earaches and all kinds of infections, bleeding.

Gelsemium (Yellow Jasmine)

This remedy is indicated in some cases of flu. Like chamomilla for teething pains, it is probably used too frequently – make sure the symptoms fit the remedy picture.

Psychological State: Nervous, perhaps trembling. Nervous about forthcoming events like exams, dental appointments or any ordeal. Tired, dull, heavy, slow, weak and sleepy. Mental paralysis from fear. Blankness of mind.

General Characteristics: Lack of thirst. Weakness: droopy eyelids or jaw. Limbs feel heavy, head needs support. Sleepy look. Weak muscles. Trembling and shivering, worse from exertion.

Modalities: Worse from bad news or excitement. Better from alcoholic drinks, conversation, and after urinating.

Causation: Warm weather after the winter. Flu in spring or autumn.

Other Features: Chills up and down the back, aches all over.

Illnesses: Mainly flu and anticipatory nervousness, but also measles, labour, headaches and diarrhoea.

Hamamelis (Witch Hazel)

Hamamelis can give temporary relief for complaints connected with the blood of veins, eg varicose veins, piles and bleeding from veins, especially in pregnancy. The affected parts are usually inflamed, sore and made worse by touch. It may be needed for nosebleeds where there is a little bleeding that will not stop; for bruising that persists after arnica and to apply to minor burns and wounds.

Hepar Sulphuris
Psychological State: Irritability arising from oversensitivity. Oversensitivity to the slightest cold, touch, pain, frustration, etc. The patient tends to be very touchy, dissatisfied and unreasonable. Fainting from pain.
General Characteristics: There is often pus involved in hepar sulph. – in throat or skin infections, gum abscesses, etc. The pus may have a bad smell. The affected part is often very sensitive to cold, draughts, touch etc. Pains as if from a splinter or fish bone.
Modalities: Worse from cold, draughts, any part of the body being uncovered, touch. Better from warmth, hot drinks, damp warmth.
Other Features: Needed sometimes for coughs: croup or croupy coughs worse in cold air. Cough with hoarseness and choking, perhaps with thick yellow mucus.
Illnesses: Coughs and all kinds of infections, usually with the formation of pus.

Ignatia (St Ignatius' Bean)
Always consider this remedy when someone is devastated by loss or other emotion.
Psychological State: Grief from a death or a relationship break up. The patient may be overcome by feelings or try to control them, but burst into sobs, or laugh then cry, or sigh frequently. Self blame. Dislike of sympathy. Self-absorption. Changeable moods.
General Characteristics: Changeable symptoms. Fainting or sleeplessness from emotions. The feeling of a lump in the throat. There can be contradictory or surprising symptoms: an empty feeling in the stomach not relieved by eating, indigestion better from eating rich foods, cough worse once the patient starts to cough etc.

Modalities: Worse from tobacco, coffee, strong smells. Better from deep breathing, swallowing. Eating can make the patient better or worse.

Causation: Grief, disappointment, fright, humiliation, being told off, worry, anger.

Other Features: Redness of one cheek. Trembling, cramps. Yawning. Nervous twitches. Tightness between chest and abdomen.

Illnesses: Usually, but not always, emotional states or illnesses brought on by emotions.

Ipecacuanha

This is a South American shrub; the word means 'the roadside plant which makes you sick'.

General Characteristics: Mainly a remedy for coughs and stomach upsets. Nausea or breathlessness accompanying any of the complaints mentioned below.

Modalities: Worse from warmth.

Causation: Punishment, too much rich food.

Other Features: Cough or asthma etc with gasping for air, choking, fast breathing, retching. Whooping cough. Constant nausea, nausea not relieved by vomiting. Bleeding, eg of nose or uterus: perhaps foamy or in flushes. Face pale or one cheek red. Cold sweat of face. Profuse saliva.

Illnesses: Asthma, bleeding, coughs, digestive problems.

Kali Carbonicum (Potash)

As an acute remedy this is required mainly for back and chest problems. All problems tend to be worse around 3am and better leaning forwards when sitting or kneeling. The back problems typically involve a feeling of weakness in the small of the back or the sensation that the back is broken, and can come on during childbirth.

Lachesis (Venom of the Bushmaster snake)

This is a fascinating medicine because characteristics of snakes appear in the symptom picture. In snakes the organs of the right side have disappeared to make the body long and thin; the provings of lachesis produce symptoms on the left side. Also in the symptom picture is sensitivity of the throat to any constriction – the snake's weak point is its throat, and it stretches to swallow things whole.

Psychological State: The patient can be very talkative, mistrustful or jealous.

General Characteristics: Complaints above the waist are worse on the left side, or start on the left and go to the right. Everything tends to be worse as the patient falls asleep, or on waking.

Modalities: Worse from tight collars (and tight waistbands), warmth.

Causation: Jealousy.

Other Features: Blueness or purpleness of affected parts. Sensation of a lump in the throat. Constriction in the throat. Swallowing is painful. Flushes of heat come up the body. Wounds that are slow to heal and turn blue.

Illnesses: Throat and ear infections, mumps, septicaemia, bleeding (of dark blood), inflamed wounds, bites and stings, food poisoning.

Lycopodium (Clubmoss)

This remedy can be needed in many different illnesses which have the two important modalities of worse at 4pm and worse on the right side.

Psychological State: Nervousness about forthcoming events or new tasks. Lack of self-confidence. A desire for company nearby but not in the same room.

General Characteristics: Desire for hot drinks, which may relieve the symptoms or make the person feel better (but sometimes the patient desires cold drinks). Hunger, with fullness after only a little food. Often indicated in digestive or liver problems where there is bloating and flatulence. Complaints which start on the right side and spread to the left.

Modalities: Worse at 4pm (or 4–8pm), on the right side, from tight clothes. Better after midnight, from passing wind.

Other Features: Yellowness of skin.

Illnesses: Infections (eg of ear, throat or chest), digestive problems, liver problems, anticipatory fears, any illness where the symptoms indicate lycopodium.

Magnesia Phosphorica (Magnesium phosphate)
A remedy for nerves and muscles, therefore often indicated in conditions such as cramps, spasms, colic and nerve pains. Heat and warm applications such as hot water bottles give relief. The pains can be sudden and violent and shoot around. Pressure on the painful place helps. This pattern could be present in period pains, sciatica, repetitive strain injury (including from playing musical instruments), toothache, etc.

Mercury
Mercury was used widely as a conventional medicine at the time when Hahnemann developed homeopathy. It was a severe treatment, often given until the patient could no longer bear the side effects, which included profuse salivation, ulcers and purging.
Psychological State: Weak and agitated, perhaps hurried. Rapid talking or stammering. Unpredictable behaviour.
General Characteristics: The mercury patient is sensitive to temperature (like thermometers, which make use of this property of mercury the metal), and is usually either too hot or too cold. Nothing seems to help except moderate temperature and rest. Complaints accompanied by excess salivation causing dribbling or dampening of the pillow. Bloody or septic discharges which may burn the skin. Offensive sweat.
Modalities: Worse from both heat and cold, at night, from perspiring.
Other Features: The mouth is often affected when mercury is needed: the tongue may be flabby and shaped at the sides by the teeth. Also possible are swollen gums, bad breath and a metallic taste in the mouth. Painful diarrhoea.
Illnesses: All kinds of infections including tonsillitis and conjunctivitis, earaches, chicken pox, mumps, swollen glands, diarrhoea, food poisoning, toothache.

Natrum Muriaticum
Potentized sodium chloride (common salt) is a more important remedy than its humble origin suggests. It is most often needed as a constitutional remedy, but heals some allergic reactions, catarrhal problems and cases of sunstroke or heat exhaustion.
    Salt controls the body's fluids. In the symptom picture there

may be dryness, for instance of the eyes, or the other extreme – streaming discharges which are watery or like egg-white. The patient is usually very thirsty, and may get worse at 10am each morning. A special feature of nat. mur. is a 'mapped' tongue, where patches of the tongue are discoloured.

Nux Vomica (Poison Nut)
This remedy is needed for all sorts of conditions.
Psychological State: A nux vom. patient tends to be bad-tempered, impatient, critical and hypersensitive. This may arise from an inner frustration with hindrances. The senses are acute and noise, smells, pain and discomfort, etc, can annoy the patient tremendously.
General Characteristics: Counter-productive efforts of body or mind, for example constipation with lots of straining, or dogged efforts to achieve misguided aims. Easily chilled.
Modalities: Worse at 3 or 4am and from cold, uncovering, or tight waistbands.
Causation: Overwork. Loss of sleep. Overindulgence in food, alcohol, coffee, drugs or medicines. Getting angry.
Other Features: Sleeplessness from overwork. Cramps, twitching and spasms: muscle spasms (eg of the back, when turning over in bed is very painful), violent vomiting, abdominal cramping pains, spasmodic cough, muscle strains from coughing or sneezing, hiccoughs, sneezing etc.
Illnesses: Back pain, sciatica, digestive problems of all kinds, coughs, asthma, fevers, hay fever, allergies, cystitis, hangovers, travel sickness and any illness which fits the nux vom. picture.

Opium (Opium Poppy)
Morphine is made from opium and is named after the Ancient Greek god of sleep, Morpheus. In material doses it suppresses pain and has a sedative effect, in smaller doses it produces dreaminess and detachment from the world.

In acute homeopathic treatment, opium is used to cure those states, whether due to a stroke, a general anaesthetic, a fright or shock, or fever. The patient is usually apathetic, with dulled senses and reduced vital activity (resulting in constipation, weak breathing, etc). There may be a glassy look in the eyes and dark red colouring of the face. High fevers that cause a state of stupor, possibly with snoring.

Petroleum (Crude Oil)

This is used as a remedy for travel sickness of car, train, boat or plane when there is also dizziness or headache. Fresh air tends to make the sickness worse.

Phosphorus

This element bursts into flame as soon as it is exposed to the air, and glows in the dark.

Psychological State: Alert and excitable, or burnt out and exhausted. Impressionable, imaginative and fearful of the dark, of being alone and about their illness etc.

General Characteristics: Acute senses. Overheated from excitement. Burning pains, eg in chest or digestive system. Desire for cold food or ice-cold drinks, but sometimes all food and drink are soon vomited. Blood-streaked vomit, mucus or diarrhoea.

Modalities: Worse from cold, change of temperature, on left side, when lying on left side, when lying on the painful side. Better after eating (the patient may be hungry even during a fever or headache), from massage.

Other Features: Profuse red bleeding, eg of nose, or from cuts. Heat located in one part of the body or rising up the back. An important remedy for many chest problems, especially left-sided pneumonia. There may be tightness of the chest and loss of voice.

Illnesses: Bleeding, coughs and chest problems, digestive problems, exhaustion, fever, nosebleeds and any illness presenting phosphorus symptoms.

Podophyllum (May Apple)

This is a remedy for diarrhoea which is worse in the morning, even as early as 4am. There may be gurgling in the abdomen leading to gushing diarrhoea which leaves the patient exhausted. This may be caused by teething or hot summer weather. Stroking the tummy helps. Diarrhoea and constipation may alternate.

Pulsatilla (the Pasque Flower, or Wind Flower)
There is a characteristic emotional state in this remedy. Consider pulsatilla in any illness when the patient is tearful and needs a lot of emotional support.
Psychological State: Uncertain and undecided, easily influenced and perhaps needing lots of reassurance, affection or physical contact. Changeable moods. The patient tends to weep easily. Clingy children.
General Characteristics: Changeable symptoms; pains may move from place to place or the nature of the complaint itself may change. Very little thirst, even though the mouth may be dry.
Modalities: Better from fresh air, sympathy, gentle movement, after crying. Worse from rich or fatty food, warmth, stuffy rooms.
Causation: After measles, after getting wet.
Other Features: Fainting from too much heat. Profuse bland catarrh.
Illnesses: This remedy can cure any kind of illness when the symptoms fit the pulsatilla picture.

Rheum (Eastern Rhubarb)
The symptom picture of this remedy can be similar to chamomilla, with its diarrhoea during teething, sour smelling discharges and bad temper. Consider it if chamomilla does not work.

Rhus Toxicodendron (Poison Ivy)
This restless trailing plant was introduced as a medicine 200 years ago when someone was accidentally poisoned by it; afterwards a blistery rash of many years duration disappeared.
    Rhus tox. in first aid treatment was described in the previous chapter; the picture is extended here.
Psychological State: Weepy, sad or restless.
General Characteristics: Restlessness, due to the fact that continued movement gives relief of body or mind. Tossing and turning: no position is comfortable. The patient may become exhausted and have to rest eventually. Desire for cold milk or other cold drinks.
Modalities: Worse when at rest, on beginning to move, from

overexertion, at night, in the autumn. Better from change of position, continued motion, warmth, a hot bath.
Causation: Exposure to cold and damp (eg camping) or getting chilled when hot.
Other Features: Redness of the tip of the tongue. Sprains and strains or exhaustion from lifting heavy things, overwork or too much exercise. Skin conditions with burning blisters or an itchy red rash. Hard swollen glands.
Illnesses: Infections and fevers including chicken pox and mumps, shingles, herpes, nappy rash, flu, sore throats, exhaustion, sprains and strains, stiffness, backache, sciatica.

Rumex
Yellow dock is a remedy for coughs which are made worse by inhaling cold air.

Sarsaparilla
Wild liquorice is a remedy for cystitis (or kidney infections) when the pain is worse at the end of urinating, when passing the last few drops. Sometimes the pains make the patient scream.

Sepia (Ink of the Cuttlefish)
This is mainly a remedy for chronic illness (see page 113), but may also be needed in pregnancy, childbirth and acute gynaecological problems. The symptom picture includes nausea from smells, especially of food. There can be pains dragging downwards in the uterus region. The person tends to feel worn out and emotionally unresponsive.

Silica
Psychological State: Resignation in the face of stress, fear of failure. Nervousness before important events.
General Characteristics: Cold, tired and weak. Sweat with an unpleasant smell, even when cold, especially on feet, head and the back of the neck. Pains as from a splinter, fish bone, needle, etc. Often given to help expel foreign bodies like splinters. Fungal infections like athlete's foot. Silica complaints tend to

come on slowly.

Modalities: Worse lying on the painful side, after drinking milk.

Causation: Vaccination, or control of a discharge or perspiration.

Other Features: Often needed for septic conditions, boils and abscesses, including those which linger on a long time. Teeth abscesses. The remedy most often needed for babies who vomit breast milk. Lumpy phlegm.

Illnesses: Ear problems, septic conditions, abscesses, some breast-feeding problems, mastitis.

Spongia

For some reason powdered burnt sponge came into use as a medicine in the Middle Ages in Europe. In homeopathy it is used mainly for coughs (usually dry coughs) with breathing difficulties, which may be made worse by exertion, excitement and after sleep. Warm food or drink may help.

Sulphur

Sulphur is one of the most widely used remedies in homeopathy. It is made from flowers of sulphur, a yellow deposit formed by volcanic eruptions. Eruptions, heat and sulphur-like smells are themes in the symptom picture.

Psychological State: Tired, lazy, messy and unconcerned.

General Characteristics: Heat, burning pains, burning discharges. Sore red lips, anus or other body orifices. Flatulence or discharges may smell of rotten eggs. Burning heat of the hands or feet, especially of the soles. A weak, hungry, empty feeling at mid-morning.

Modalities: Worse at 10–12am, from warmth, washing or bathing, while standing.

Other Features: Diarrhoea that forces the patient to get out of bed in the morning.

Illnesses: Any illness presenting the sulphur symptom picture.

Staphysagria (Stavesacre or Larkspur, a delphinium)

Needed in many complaints that arise from suppressed emotions, especially unexpressed anger. The person may feel humiliated, invaded or abused and not be able to do anything about it. Trembling with emotion. Nerves may be hypersensitive.

This remedy is sometimes needed for painful wounds, after surgery (especially if a body opening has been stretched) and in cystitis connected with sexual intercourse.

Tabacum
Tobacco is used to treat some cases of travel sickness, and nausea in pregnancy. With the nausea there may be paleness of the face and sweating. Cool air helps.

Urtica Urens
This remedy has been described in the first aid chapter. It is also required sometimes for hives or prickly heat – and it may regulate the supply of breast milk, when there is too little *or* too much, if no other remedy is indicated by the symptoms.

10

Constitutional Treatment and Developing Your Skills

IN CONVENTIONAL MEDICINE most chronic, or long-term, ill-nesses are regarded as incurable. The treatment is directed towards controlling the symptoms. Homeopathy has a lot to offer because successful treatment can achieve profound trans-formations in health.

When you have learnt how to treat acute, or short-term, con-ditions then go on to begin treating some chronic conditions.

EXTENDING YOUR SKILLS TO TREAT CHRONIC ILLNESS

Chronic and constitutional treatment are the same thing. Chronic illnesses arise from the constitution, that is, the psycho-logical and physical type of the patient, and it is this which must be treated. Sometimes constitutional treatment is given when the patient is not particularly ill to prevent illness and to boost general health and well-being.

Chapter 4, 'Your Visit to a Homeopath', gives some insights into a consultation for constitutional treatment. Much of what you have learned for acute treatment in chapter 6 still applies. A crucial difference is in the case-taking, (stage two of homeo-pathic treatment, see the beginning of chapter 6). The constitu-tional case-taking extends backwards in time and into the personality and daily life of the patient.

Begin by recording all you can discover about the health problems which the patient first mentions. Ask if there is anything else, letting the patient know that stresses and emotional problems can be included. When you have explored all these issues then check that the following topics have been covered:

- how the illness (or illnesses) began, and whether any stress or trauma was a trigger;
- at some stage in the consultation find out about any difficult phases, stresses or traumas that have affected the patient deeply at any time, from birth onwards;
- medical history from birth to the present, including treatments of all kinds;
- reactions to weather conditions, climate changes, seasons, open air and stuffy rooms, etc;
- variations in symptoms, energy and mood according to time of day or night;
- appetite, thirst, food likes and dislikes, and any foods which cause bad effects;
- the quality and pattern of the patient's sleep, including the times of waking and the state of mind; also any recurring dreams;
- for women, any problems associated with the menstrual cycle;
- the emotional characteristics of the person such as anxieties, fears, depression, apathy, nervousness, irritability or anger;
- the patient's responses to others – family, friends, colleagues and strangers;
- problems with memory, concentration, understanding, etc.

This list is given to suggest areas for exploration. You can use each item as a starting point and let the patient respond. Follow the patient's lead unless he or she is going off the subject altogether. When a line of enquiry ends, go back to the list. Your notes will stray away from the order above if you are building up a living image of the patient and how he or she functions in daily life.

As always, a homeopath tries to stick to open-ended questions, and to be sensitive to any hints from the patient, conscious or unconscious, of areas which should be explored. Simply asking patients to give a personality sketch of themselves can be very helpful. Record your own impressions of the person.

USING HOMEOPATHIC REMEDIES FOR CHRONIC ILLNESS

Professional Help: Most patients in this category have already been to their doctor, know the diagnosis and may be taking orthodox medicines. You should recommend many of them to see a professional homeopath.

Do not treat any patients who are chronically weak, very elderly or seriously ill. If you decide to treat a chronic skin condition stick to the potencies 6x, 12x and 6c to minimize any aggravation. Remember that oral steroids or antibiotics usually antidote homeopathic treatment.

Dose: One tablet of low potency 3 times a day for 3 days, or *one dose* of potency 30. Always stop the treatment as soon as there is any change in the condition.

Assessment: Assess the effects of the low potencies 3 days after the treatment is over. Assess potency 30 after 4–6 weeks. With the higher potencies it is sometimes several weeks before the remedy starts to work and patience is needed. If there is no improvement after these waiting times then give a new remedy.

If there is an improvement, wait. Repeat the same remedy later if the improvement wears off. Patience may be needed here too because, in this category, repeating the medicine at the wrong time or giving a new one can make the treatment ineffective. Do not repeat the treatment for slight or temporary relapses. This is one of the common mistakes in homeopathy.

To work out the remedy the guidance in chapter 6 in the section 'Working Out The Remedy' is indispensable. You will also need assistance from some of the books listed in the appendix. Don't give the remedy there and then – think about it for a few days to help get things in perspective.

USING THE RECOMMENDED BOOKS

A student of homeopathy studies homeopathic methods and principles, the remedy pictures (materia medica), and needs to know how to make good use of a repertory. This is all cemented together by actual experience with patients. This book and the introductory books in the appendix include something of all these; you can begin to treat chronic problems with these introductory books. The advanced books are more specialized and each covers one aspect only, so a serious student needs at least three textbooks: a *how to do it* book, a *repertory* and a *materia medica*. The first tells you, among other things, how to use the repertory and materia medica. After taking the case and putting the symptoms in order, you use the repertory to arrive at a short list of possible remedies. You then study these in the materia medica to make the final choice.

To a certain extent the choice of books is a matter of personal preference. However, if you want to put some serious time and study into homeopathy, you will find it hard to do without *The Science of Homeopathy*, Kent's *Repertory*, or one of the expanded versions of it, and Phatak's *Materia Medica*.

A student must learn about the human body and its diseases. In addition to a first aid manual and a family health guide consider getting a medical text book.

FURTHER TRAINING

Try to go to an evening class or an introductory course. This adds another dimension to your learning process.

All this involves an escalating commitment of time and money which could culminate in a professional training. If you want to become either a professional homeopath or spend some years studying, details of colleges are available from the professional societies listed at the back of this book. Short of that, homeopathy is still a very rewarding interest which benefits others and you can select your own level of involvement. A lot can be achieved just with this book and a few remedies.

GENERAL GUIDANCE ON CONSTITUTIONAL TREATMENT

When a constitutional treatment is working several things, apart from a straightforward improvement, can happen.

- There can be an aggravation of the symptoms at first.
- The patient may feel better before the health problems themselves improve.

- Some of the problems may take longer to get better than others.
- Old symptoms may return briefly.
- A rash or discharge can appear.

To get the best from homeopathy it is important not to give more remedies or other new treatments while these changes are taking place.

I have just treated two people for ME. They were gradually improving, and then they developed colds like those they had had several years previously at the beginning of their illnesses. This time the colds were short and mild, and were a stage on the journey in the opposite direction. Afterwards, their rate of recovery accelerated.

The temporary return of old symptoms is a good sign and should not be treated. Where there has been a descent into poor health through a series of illnesses, homeopathy can reverse the whole process. The remedy is working holistically, deep within the organism, beyond the level of just one of the diseases. Experiencing homeopathy at work is an education in the true nature of health and disease, and in the nature of the intelligence that the vital energy possesses.

THE LAW OF CURE

Dr Constantine Hering was a homeopath in the United States in the 19th century. His greatest contribution to medicine is called *the law of cure* and provides a yardstick to assess the overall effectiveness of any kind of treatment. After years of observing patterns of illness in thousands of people over whole lifetimes, Dr Hering saw a progression. If your health is deteriorating, you may find not only that one disease is getting worse, you may also develop new diseases. A common progression in childhood is from eczema to asthma. Conventional medicine also accepts this particular progression. The state of disease has spread from the skin into the respiratory system. Hering's Law tells us that since the lungs are more internal and are more important in the preservation of life than the skin, health in such an event has deteriorated.

This is a statement of Hering's Law: when illness progresses from a less important to a more important organ, or inwards into the organism, then the patient is getting worse, and the treatment is harmful. If the complaints are going in the opposite direction, or in the reverse order of their appearance, then the patient is improving, the treatment is doing good work, and the process must be allowed to continue undisturbed. The body has a natural tendency to cure itself by pushing its problems outwards as discharges or skin eruptions. You can observe this in the childhood illnesses. Many of the worst cases develop if the rash fails to appear properly. These illnesses usually improve once the rash appears. In measles, for example, the virus is killed in the skin rash.

By taking a full medical history homeopaths track patterns of health carefully. We often see the law of cure operating in our patients: a child's asthma will get better when the eczema he or she had as a toddler reappears. The treatment will then go on to cure the eczema too. Sometimes the same thing happens when treating hyperactivity, and other conditions.

Hippocrates, the father of Western medicine, wrote: 'In those suffering from depression of spirits and kidney disease the appearance of haemorrhoids is a good sign.'

There are very few of these standard patterns of progression. The journey of deterioration and improvement tends to be highly individual, depending on each person's susceptibility (see chapter 2).

These curative reactions are usually mild and trouble free. Homeopaths welcome them because they are followed by long periods of good health. Patients need reassurance that all is well and are usually already feeling better in themselves. It is important not to interfere by giving any new treatment, homeopathic or otherwise, to control these symptoms.

SOME CONSTITUTIONAL TYPES

Here are two examples of the dozens of common homeopathic constitutional types.

Argentum Nitricum
About half the patients who come to me because of panic

111

attacks do well on this remedy. It is silver nitrate, a substance used in photographic films because it takes the impression of light and stores the image. The patient is also impressionable – the kind of thoughts and fears that we can all have briefly and soon forget, stay in the mind of the *argentum nitricum* person and generate tremendous fear.

Along with several other remedy types they can become very nervous before an examination, a visit to the dentist or doctor, or any unusual event or anything which seems like an ordeal. This can combine with claustrophobia or agoraphobia, or sometimes both at once, to make visits to supermarkets, driving on motorways (or even on quiet roads in extreme cases) and using lifts and tube trains impossible. Other examples of situations which can induce awful panic are queues, theatres and cinemas and travel in any kind of vehicle.

Some of the fears and phobias can be more unusual. The person can start to imagine all sorts of unlikely possibilities. The first case study in chapter 4 illustrates this. The patient would lie in bed at night wondering if a plane flying over would fall out of the sky onto her. Other strange thoughts of this kind are: 'What if I were to jump out of this window? What if this building falls on me?' Life becomes very difficult when irrational thoughts like this stay on a person's mind.

No one person is going to have all these problems, but they are all symptoms which have been cured by *argentum nitricum* in different cases.

Actors and singers with stage fright or voice and throat problems may need this remedy. Diarrhoea often accompanies the nervousness before important events.

When healthy, this constitutional type is cheerful and extrovert. They love company, are lively and dynamic and can do a lot of rushing around. Their excitability and impulsiveness are positive qualities but can lead to exhaustion.

They are usually warm-blooded people who need fresh air. They often crave salty foods and sweet things. The latter can cause bloating and flatulence. Not all *arg. nit.* types will have the psychological patterns described above: the physical problems can be dizziness, catarrh, ulcers, diseases of the nervous system, eye diseases, etc.

Sepia

This remedy is made from the ink of the cuttlefish. It was first used by Hahnemann himself after he met an artist who was using sepia paints. The artist had the habit of licking his brush and the symptoms this was causing gave us our first knowledge of *sepia* as a homeopathic remedy.

Young *sepia* people are lively and excitable and often love dancing. However, when older or in poor health, their energy drops both emotionally and physically. They can be undermined by the emotional demands of their family. They feel drained and unresponsive. The needs of their children and loved ones become a burden to them. They may need to be on their own and dislike sympathy, as it requires a response, and can be irritable if disturbed.

In *sepia* women the hormonal system can easily be thrown out of balance. There can be all kinds of period, premenstrual and menopausal problems involving vaginal discharges, bearing down pains, prolapses, heavy and prolonged periods, mood changes and exhaustion. *Sepia* is one of the main homeopathic types who can suffer ill-effects from pregnancy, childbirth and oral contraceptives – all things which affect the hormonal system.

Two of the personal features which can confirm that *sepia* is the right remedy are a desire for pickles or vinegar, and a love of dancing or strenuous exercise. Despite the fact that they may be exhausted they can enjoy exertion because this seems to lift them out of their lethargy. They may also prefer to keep busy because they feel worse once they stop.

These descriptions concentrate on the personality type of the remedies because that is what is most important in selecting constitutional treatment.

11

Conclusion

THOSE WHO HAVE experienced homeopathy working respect and support it. Those who have not are often sceptical and can be totally dismissive. But outright condemnation is decreasing as surveys reveal how widely it is used and how widely its effectiveness is acknowledged. The facts speak for themselves.

Are you now fired by enthusiasm for homeopathy or awed by its complexity? Do you intend to buy all the books and remedies as soon as you can? Or are you uncertain even about taking *arnica* next time you hurt yourself?

After twelve years in full-time practice I am still fascinated by homeopathy and impressed by its power. It is a genuine source of healing. It can amaze people who are new to it, and to dedicated study it gives generous rewards.

This book is quite technical in places, especially in chapter 6. This is necessary because, like any powerful tool, homeopathy must be used properly. And to adjust our way of looking at disease to take on the homeopathic view takes time. In a way, it turns our notions of health and illness upside down.

Homeopathy is mysterious and yet profoundly practical. Every theory is rooted in observation and every attempt to work out the right remedy receives its acid test when the remedy is given to the patient.

The convenience of keeping and using homeopathic remedies at home means that many households now have some of them, usually *arnica* and a few others. The benefits are not confined to minor ailments. In many cases of serious disease homeopathic remedies offer one of the best chances of real help.

Conclusion

The future for homeopathy looks bright. The approach to health and degree of effectiveness it offers are attracting more and more people, and the demand will continue to increase. In the health revolution that is taking place homeopathy has a central role.

Notes

1 Kleinen, Knipschild et al, *Clinical Trials of Homeopathy*, British Medical Journal, London, February 1991, no 302, pp 316–23.
2 Larry Dossey, MD, *Beyond Illness*, New Science Library (Shambala), Boston, 1984, p 85.
3 Lewis Thomas, *The Medusa And The Snail*, Viking Press, London, 1974, p 94.
4 Richard Selzer, *Confessions of a Knife*, Paladin (Triad Granada), London, 1982.
5 George Vithoulkas, *The Science of Homeopathy*, Thorsons, London, 1986, p 59.
6 C G Jung, *The Psychology of the Child Archetype*, Collected Works 9i (pp 149–181), Routledge Kegan Paul, London, 1940, p 173.
7 From 'Healing' by D H Lawrence, *The Complete Poems of D H Lawrence*, by kind permission of Laurence Pollinger and the Estate of Frieda Lawrence Ravagli
8 Fritjof Capra, *The Tao of Physics*, Bantam, New York, 1977, p 211.
9 David Bohn, *Wholeness And The Implicate Order*, Routledge Kegan Paul, London, 1980, p 191.

Appendix

TESTS SHOWING THE EFFECTIVENESS OF HOMEOPATHY

In the *British Medical Journal* (1943 (ii), page 654) Florey reported that penicillin has effects in dilutions of one part in 250 million (which is like putting one drop of water in 18,000 bottles of whisky!)

In the *Journal of the American Institute of Homeopathy* (1966, no. 59, p 287, and 1968, no. 61, pp 28–9) Anna K Wannamaker shows that homeopathic potencies affected the growth rates of onion seedlings.

Professor Jacques Benveniste's research at the French government research centre INSERM in Paris was published in the scientific journal *Nature* in June 1988. It reported on experiments repeated in three countries which showed that homeopathic dilutions work.

The veterinary surgeon Christopher Day reported in the *British Homeopathic Journal* in January 1986 (no. 75 pp 11–15) that caulophyllum 30c reduced stillbirths in pigs. Christopher Day also featured in a BBC *Horizon* programme which showed herds of cows getting far less mastitis as a result of homeopathic treatment.

A trial of a homeopathic potency of pollen in treating hay fever proved that the remedy was six times better than a placebo. (Reilly, Taylor, McSharry and Aitchison; *The Lancet*, 18 October 1986, pp 881–6).

Many more examples are quoted in *Homeopathy: Medicine of the Twenty-First Century* by Dana Ullman (North Atlantic Books, California, 1988) and in *Homeopathic Science And Modern Medicine* by Harris Coulter (North Atlantic Books, California, 1980).

Glossary

>: made better by (for example, *sore throat* > *hot drinks* means that the patient's sore throat is relieved by drinking something hot).

<: made worse by.

Acute: An acute illness is a short term illness like a cold, a digestive upset or pneumonia. An acute illness can be mild or severe.

Aggravation: A temporary worsening of symptoms after taking a homeopathic remedy.

Allopathic Medicine: Orthodox medicine is allopathic, ie, it uses medicines with effects opposite to the illness.

Antidote: Something which stops homeopathic remedies working. The main examples are coffee and camphor, eucalyptus or menthol. (See chapter 5)

Case-taking: The recording of all the information about a patient which a homeopath needs.

Centesimal: The scale of potencies which is diluted to one part in a hundred at each stage of **potentisation**.

Characteristic Symptoms: Symptoms which are typical of a certain remedy, for example the slow functioning of a *gelsemium* patient.

Chronic: Chronic illnesses are long term illnesses like eczema and cancer, as opposed to **acute** illnesses.

Common Symptoms: These symptoms are usually found with a certain disease, for example a cough during a chest infection. They are of little importance in selecting the homeopathic remedy.

Constitutional Treatment: This is treatment of the whole person for long-term health problems.

Conventional Medicine: The mainstream medicine of our times, ie, **allopathic medicine**.

Decimal: The scale of potencies which are diluted to one part in ten at each stage of **potentisation**.

Defence Mechanism: The ability of a living organism to resist illness and maintain health, This includes, but is more than, the immune system.

Expectoration: The coughing up of mucus.

Flatulence: Gases in the digestive system.

General Symptoms: Symptoms of the whole person. When explaining them a patient will say, for example '*I* ache all over," rather than 'My legs ache.' Aching all over is a general symptom and is more important in choosing the homeopathic remedy. A symptom of the legs or any one part of the body is a *particular* symptom.

Immune System: The system in the body which fights infection.

Law of Cure: A medical law formulated by Dr Constantine Hering in the nineteenth century. Briefly, it states that healing begins within the patient and works its way outwards. (See chapter 10)

Law of Similarity: This states that a substance which can cause a certain set of symptoms in a healthy person can, when given in the appropriate way, cure that set of symptoms in a sick person.

Materia Medica: This latin term is used to refer to the **symptom picture** of a remedy and to the books which describe the symptom pictures of homeopathic remedies.

Modality: Anything which makes a symptom, or the whole patient, better or worse. (See < and > at the beginning of this glossary)

Mucus Membranes: The 'inner skin' or linings of the body, such as the surfaces of the lungs and digestive system.

Orifices: The openings of the body, eg, mouth, anus, etc.

Orthodox Medicine: See **Allopathic Medicine** and **Conventional Medicine**.

Placebo: A treatment which contains no medicine, eg, unmedicated pills.

Polychrest: A term used in homeopathy to describe a remedy which may be needed for many different kinds of illness.

Potency: The potency of a homeopathic remedy is the number of times it has been potentised (see below).

Potentisation: The process of preparing a homeopathic medicine by repeated methodical dilution and shaking.

Proving: The testing of homeopathic medicines on human volunteers.

Relapse: Getting worse again after getting better.

Remedy: The term used most often to refer to a homeopathic medicine.

Remedy Picture: The result of the **proving** of a homeopathic remedy. The remedy picture includes all the symptoms which a remedy can cause and cure – far more symptoms than any one patient will ever have. The remedy picture (or symptom picture) also conveys the character and the themes of the remedy, which are patterns in the symptoms. These make the remedy pictures much easier to understand and remember.

Repertory: A book or part of a book which is an index of symptoms. After each symptom is a list of all the remedies which may cure that symptom. By cross-referencing the one remedy which covers the whole symptom picture can be found. This cross-referencing is called *repertorisation*.

Rubric: A symptom listed in a repertory.

Sac lac: Milk sugar, the usual substance used as the base for homeopathic tablets.

Similarity: See **Law of Similarity**.

Similimum: The latin term for the similar remedy, ie, the correct homeopathic remedy.

Succusion: The shaking process used in **potentisation**.

Suppression: The control, or driving inwards, of symptoms or illnesses.

Susceptibility: Vulnerability, or openness to, illness or things which can cause illness. This is caused by a flawed defence mechanism in the patient.

Symptom: Any disturbance of healthy functioning. Symptoms can be classified in many ways eg, whether they are **general** or particular, by their severity and according to disease categories.

Symptom Picture: All the important symptoms of a patient (or of a remedy) stated in such a way as to convey the nature of the patient (or remedy).

Tinctures: Unpotentised medicines in liquid form. They are used as the starting point for potentisation, or sometimes diluted 5 drops per tablespoon to make a lotion for external applications (eg calendula).

Vital Energy: The energy of living things which maintains life and health, and heals wounds and disease. Homeopathic remedies stimulate the vital energy.

Remedy Abbreviations

Abbreviation	Latin name	Common name
Acon.	Aconitum Napellus	Aconite
All. cep.	Allium Cepa	Red Onion
Ant. tart.	Antimonium Tartaricum	Tartar Emetic
Apis (apis mel.)	Apis Mellifica	Honey Bee
Arn.	Arnica Montana	The Fall Herb
Ars. (ars. alb.)	Arsenicum Album	White Arsenic
Bell.	Belladonna	Deadly Nightshade
Bellis	Bellis Perennis	Daisy
Bry.	Bryonia	White Bryony
Cal.	Calendula Officinalis	Small Marigold
Canth.	Cantharis	Spanish Fly
Carbo veg.	Carbo Vegetabilis	Wood Charcoal
Caust.	Causticum	Caustic Potash
Cham.	Chamomilla Matricaria	German Chamomile
Cina.	Cina Officinalis	Wormseed
Coff.	Coffea Tosta	Roasted Coffee
Coloc.	Colocynthis	Bitter Cucumber
Dros.	Drosera Rotundifolia	Sundew
Eup. perf.	Eupatorium Perfoliata	Boneset
Euphr.	Euphrasia	Eyebright
Ferr. phos.	Ferrum Phosphoricum	Iron Phosphate
Gels.	Gelsemium Sempervirens	Yellow Jasmine
Ham.	Hamamelis	Witch Hazel
Hep. (Hep. Sulph.)	Hepar Sulphuris Calcareum	Calcium Sulphide
Hyp.	Hypericum Perfoliatum	St John's Wort
Ign.	Ignatia Amara	St Ignatius' Bean
Ipec.	Ipecacuanha	——
Kali Bich.	Kali Bichromicum	Potassium Bichromate

Kali Carb.	Kali Carbonicum	Potassium Carbonate
Lach.	Lachesis	Venom of Bushmaster Snake
Led.	Ledum Palustre	Marsh Tea
Lyc.	Lycopodium Clavatum	Club Moss
Mag. Phos.	Magnesia Phosphorica	Magnesium Phosphate
Merc. (Merc. Sol.)	Mercurius Solubilis	Mercury (Quicksilver)
Nat. Mur.	Natrum Muriaticum	Common Salt
Nux Vom.	Nux Vomica	Poison Nut
Op.	Opium	Juice of White Poppy
Petr.	Petroleum	Crude Oil
Phos.	Phosphorus	White Phosphorus
Podo.	Podophyllum	May Apple
Puls.	Pulsatilla Nigricans	Wind Flower (Pasque Flower)
Rad. Brom.	Radium Bromide	———
Rheum	Rheum	Eastern Rhubarb
Rhus Tox.	Rhus Toxicondendron	Poison Ivy
Rumex.	Rumex Crispus	Yellow Dock
Ruta.	Ruta Graveolens	Common Rue
Sars.	Sarsaparilla	Wild Liquorice
Sep.	Sepia	Ink of the Cuttlefish
Sil.	Silica	Flint (Rock Crystal)
Spong.	Spongia Tosta	Roasted Sponge
Sulph.	Sulphur	Flowers of Sulphur
Staph.	Staphysagria	Stavesacre
Symph.	Symphytum	Comfrey
Tabac.	Tabacum	Tobacco
Urt. (Urt Urens)	Urtica Urens	Dwarf Stinging Nettle

Further Reading

Homeopathy: Medicine of the New Man by George Vithoulkas (Thorsons, England, 1985) An inspiring read by one of the world's leading homeopaths.

INTRODUCTORY BOOKS

The Complete Homeopathy Handbook by Miranda Castro (Macmillan, England, 1990) Similar to *Health Essentials: Homeopathy* in its subject matter, but larger and more comprehensive.

The Complete Family Guide by Dr Christopher Hammond (Element Books, 1995) An illustrated introductory book.

ADVANCED BOOKS

The Science of Homeopathy by George Vithoulkas (Thorsons, England, 1986) An essential textbook.

Homeopathy as Art And Science by Dr Elizabeth Wright Hubbard (Beaconsfield Publishers) This selection of writings includes *A Brief Study Course In Homeopathy* which is excellent.

Homeopathic Drug Pictures by Margaret Tyler (Health Science Press, England, 1970) A lively and thorough materia medica of over 100 homeopathic remedies.

Materia Medica of Homeopathic Medicines by S R Phatak (Indian Books and Periodicals Syndicae) A good reference book used by many homeopaths on a daily basis.

Repertory of the Homeopathic Materia Medica by James Tyler Kent. This repertory, or one of the modern versions which include important additional material, is essential for a serious student.

Emotional Healing with Homeopathy by Peter Chappell (Element Books, 1993) This book explains self-help for emotional problems and connects homeopathy with psychotherapy.

Useful Addresses

HOMEOPATHIC RESOURCES IN THE UK AND IRELAND

Professional homeopaths (R S Hom) are represented and regulated by *The Society of Homeopaths*, 2 Artizan Road, Northampton NN1 4HU. Tel: 01604 21400. Information on colleges providing training in homeopathy can also be obtained from this society. The equivalent body in Ireland is *The Irish Society of Homeopaths* 32 Strand Street, Cloghae Head, Co. Louth. Tel: 041 22702.

Doctor homeopaths (M F Hom) have trained in homeopathy and become members of the Faculty of Homeopathy. Contact: *The British Homeopathic Association*, 27a Devonshire Street, London W1N 1RJ. Tel: 0171 935 2163.

Suppliers of homeopathic books
Some books are available from local book shops. Otherwise contact: Minerva Books Mail Order Service, 6 Bothwell St, London W6 8DY. Tel: 0171 385 2182.

Suppliers of homeopathic remedies
Ainsworths Homeopathic Pharmacy, 3 New Cavendish Street, London W1M 7LH. Tel: 0171 935 5330 and 0171 487 5253.
Galen Homeopathic Pharmacy, Lewel Mill, West Stafford, Dorchester, Dorset DT2 8AN. Tel: 01305 263996.
Helios Homeopathic Pharmacy, 97 Camden Road, Tunbridge Wells, Kent TN1 2QP. Tel: 01892 537254 and 536393.

Nelson and Co. Ltd, Customer Services, 5 Endeavour Way, London SW19 9UH. Tel: 0181 946 8527.

Weleda (UK) Ltd, Heanor Road, Ilkeston, Derbyshire DE7 8DR. Tel: 01602 303151.

HOMEOPATHIC RESOURCES IN THE USA

The National Center for Homeopathy can inform you of homeopaths (doctors and other professionals) in your area. The center also publishes a newsletter and provides educational programs etc. The address is 801 N. Fairfax Street, Suite 306, Alexandria, Virginia 22314. Phone: 703 548 7790.

Suppliers of homeopathic remedies
Boericke and Tafel, 2381 Circadian Way, Santa Rosa, CA 95407. Tel: 707 571 8202.

Boiron-Bornemann, 6 Campus Blvd, Newtown Square, PA 19073. Tel: 610 325 7464.

Dolisos, 3014 Rigel Ave, Las Vegas, NV 89102. Tel: 800 365 4767.

Longevity Pure Medicines, 9595 Wilshire Blvd *502, Beverly Hills. CA 90212. Tel: 310 273 7423.

Standard Homeopathic Co, 210 W 131st St, Los Angeles, CA 90061. Tel: 800 624 9659.

Washington Homeopathic Products, 124 Fairfax St, Berkeley Springs, WV 25411. Tel: 304 258 2541.

You can get a list of manufacturers of homeopathic medicines from *The Homeopathic Pharmacopoeia Convention of the US*, 1500 Massachusetts Ave. NW., *41, Washington DC 20005 or from *The American Association of Homeopathic Pharmacies* PO Box 2273, Falls Church, Virginia VA 22042. Tel: 703-532 3237.

Suppliers of homeopathic books
(and information on homeopathy): Homeopathic Educational Services, 2124 Kittredge St., Berkeley, CA 94704. Tel: 510-649 0294.

Useful Addresses

HOMEOPATHIC RESOURCES IN CANADA

Canadian Society of Homeopaths, 87 Meadowland Drive West, Nepean, Ontario K2G2R9.
Vancouver Centre for Homeopathy, 2246 Spruce St, Vancouver, BC, V6H 2P3.

HOMEOPATHIC RESOURCES IN AUSTRALIA

The Australian Federation of Homeopaths, PO Box 806, Spit Junction, New South Wales 2088.
Australian Association of Professional Homeopaths, PO Box 4052, Daisy Hill 4127, Queensland.
Australian Institute of Homeopathy, 21 Bulah Close, Berowra Heights, New South Wales 2082.
Brauer Biotherapies (Pharmacy), 1 Para Rd., Tanunda, S. Australia 5352.
Society of Classical Homeopaths, 2nd Floor, Paxton House, 90 Pilt St, Sydney 2000.

HOMEOPATHIC RESOURCES IN NEW ZEALAND

Institute of Classical Homeopathy, 24 West Haven Drive, Tawa, Wellington, New Zealand. Tel: 6443 28051.
Len Hooper Pharmacy, 104 Oxford Terrace, Epuni, Lower Hutt. Tel: 04 567 7199.
The New Zealand Homeopathic Society, PO Box 67-095, Mount Eden, Auckland 3.

HOMEOPATHIC RESOURCES IN AFRICA

Homeopathic Society of South Africa, PO Box 9658, Johannesburg 2000.
African Homeopathic Medical Foundation, PO Box 131, Nempi, Oru LGA, Imo State, Nigeria.
W Last Pharmacy, PO Box 407, Johannesburg 2000. Tel: 011 680 5580.

Index

Index